"After two decades of buying expensive beauty products, I am s⟨...⟩ are friendly to the environment and safe for my skin. I am amaz⟨...⟩ ⟨...⟩ in just three short weeks and will continue to use Dr. Daniels' simple and affordable regimen. Thank you, Dr. Ray, for sharing this valuable information with all of us."

—Heidi Beard, Gig Harbor, WA

"It has been over ten years now since I received a riveting diagnosis of hepatitis C. In that moment, I decided that it would not win. I took charge of my health, committing to nutritional and lifestyle changes that would allow me to avoid pharmaceutical treatment if at all possible. Cleansing with fasts and colonics was an obvious way to support my liver. Little did I know that the changes I was making in order to survive would reward me with increased energy and radiant skin. What might have killed me has made me more beautiful.

"My viral load that first numbered over a million was last read at 7,500. I attribute this to listening carefully each day to what my body needs and wants. I have found Do you have the guts to be beautiful? to be a loving adjunct to this daily dialogue. Like Drs. Ray and Daniels in their helpful guidebook, may we each claim an outer beauty—for ourselves and for our planet—that comes from deep within."

—Patricia Cannon Childs, Nashville, TN

"I have spent over 30 years searching for 'simple' health. My diet has always been a challenge to me, and I would frequently experience fatigue, bloating, and indigestion after meals.

"Thanks to whole food nutrition, the Green Drink, and the liver flush, I have never felt more alive and energized! I appreciate the weight loss as well—14 pounds in the first 35 days! My husband, Darrell, lost 16 pounds during the 10-day liver flush, and a total of 23 pounds in the first 35 days, even though he couldn't be totally faithful during his travels.

"The natural beauty regimes are not only easy and fun, they're inexpensive. I threw away all of my expensive non-edible makeup, and my skin is glowing!

"Thank you to Drs. Ray and Daniels for sharing this timely, 'self-care' message with everyone. You have truly blessed your readers!"

—Judy Strickler, R.N., Clovis, CA

"The definition of beauty has eluded scholars, poets, mathematicians, writers, and the average person on the street ever since time began. The reason is that beauty is an holistic gestalt that is understood by our right brain (the artistic brain), but yet, we ask our left brain (the analytical brain) to describe it.

"Creating beauty is even more elusive, as can be witnessed by the plethora of treatments and procedures out there. Yet even with such intervention, very few patients actually look more beautiful. They simply look more 'done.'

"The first step to understanding the complex nature of beauty is to recognize that not one person in human history has ever been made more beautiful by the removal of a single wrinkle or a solitary blemish. In Do you have the guts to be beautiful?, Drs. Daniels and Ray have gone well beyond that first step. They not only understand that beauty is actually a sign of inner health, but also that inner health is reflected in the only areas of our body exposed to the outside world—namely, our skin and hair.

"Giving the gift of inner health to ourselves sends the subconscious messages to the world around us, and more importantly, to ourselves, that we are indeed beautiful—and we will have the glow to prove it.

"In their first book, Drs. Daniels and Ray have managed to bring the two sides of the brain—the artistic and the analytical—just a bit closer to each other. I look forward to passing on their insightful and very practical advice to my patients and family alike."

—Frederick A. Coville, M.D.
Plastic and Reconstructive Surgeon
Worldwide Lecturer on Skin and Beauty
London and New Jersey

Do you have the guts to be beautiful?

JENNIFER DANIELS, M.D.

AND

MITRA RAY, PH.D.

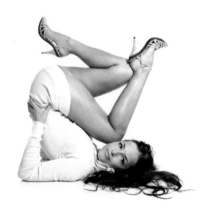

SHINING STAR MEDIA

MARYSVILLE, WASHINGTON

Printed in the United States of America

Publisher's Cataloging-In-Publication Data

Daniels, Jennifer, 1957-
   Do you have the guts to be beautiful? / Jennifer Daniels and Mitra Ray. -- Limited 1st ed.

   p. : ill. ; cm.

   Includes bibliographical references and index.
   ISBN: 978-0-9714342-1-9

1. Skin--Care and hygiene. 2. Skin--Aging. 3. Beauty, Personal. 4. Aging--Nutritional aspects. I. Ray, Mitra. II. Title.

RL87 .D36 2009
646.7/26   2008939972

Design by Jill Byrd Williams

Shining Star Media
P.O. Box 383
Marysville, Washington 98270
www.DrMitraRay.com

To all those who want to be beautiful,
and honor our beautiful home, Mother Earth

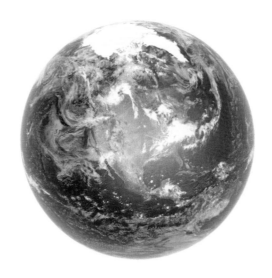

Table of Contents

FIGURES

TABLES

HELPFUL RESOURCES

At the end of this book, you'll find a list of suggested readings, resources for purchasing suggested therapeutic items, as well as a bibliography, containing references cited in the text.

ACKNOWLEDGMENTS

I would like to acknowledge my mother and my daughters who agreeably tried the natural concoctions that I devised to erase acne, wrinkles, and gray hair. I would also like to acknowledge my patients for patiently and persistently telling me how they valued their looks above all else. Finally I listened, and this book was born. To all the gorgeous people I have met who showed me that one does not have to become gray and wrinkled with age – thank you.

—Jennifer Daniels, M.D.

I am grateful to my loving husband, Doug, for supporting me in every way. He has been a willing subject of my experimentation over the years, including facials, Green Drinks and liver flushes! I have no words for the inspiration I receive from my two beautiful daughters—and they too share my spirit of exploration. I am blessed with more than my share of friends and family who love and support me: Dipankar, Kelly, Gayle, John, JoAnn, Patricia, my family in India, and so, so many other friends, especially in the world of NSA/Juice Plus+®. A special thanks to my editors Kelly Koffman and Patricia Cannon Childs. And to my growing list of mentors, including Prof. T. Colin Campbell and Dr. Jennifer Daniels, thank you for being so willing to share your knowledge with me and with the world.

—Mitra Ray, Ph.D.

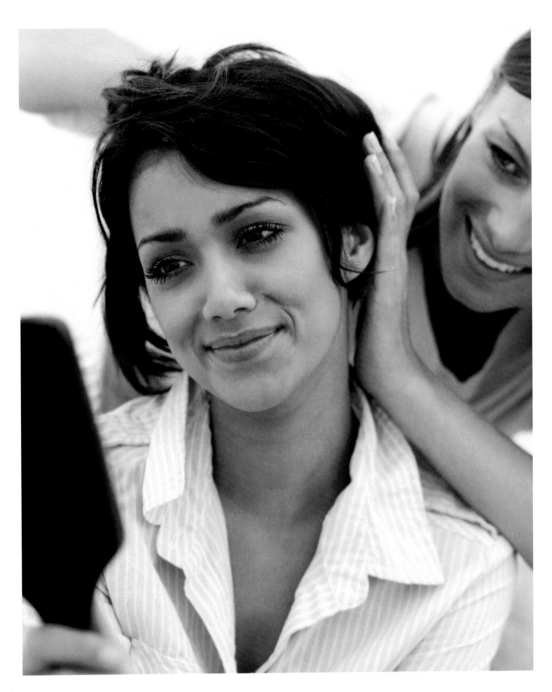

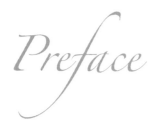

Preface

Reading this book may alter the very way in which you look in the mirror, and provide you with more detail than even your doctor can get from the fanciest and most expensive tests. This doesn't mean that you no longer need to see a doctor; rather, it means that your face can provide you with a wealth of empowering information. We'll share some little-known miracles of the body and, specifically, how your face tells a story of what is happening inside you. After reading this book, you'll be able to unlock the messages your face is giving you; you'll learn simple, yet effective steps that you can take to look and feel better – sans pills, chemicals, or complicated recipes.

Unfortunately, a trip to the doctor can't make you look younger or heal you unless you begin to make lifestyle changes. Change is hard. It's hard for pets and small children, and it's no different for us. Just try moving to a new house, and you'll see how much your pet loves that! Or displace a wild animal, and chances are that it will die.

Humans also resist change. Nevertheless, what's the benefit of making changes? If you should choose this book as a guide and adopt the suggested practices, not only will you physically begin to take decades off of your appearance, but you will also feel terrific!

Not too long ago, I had the absolute pleasure of meeting Dr. Jennifer Daniels during a health retreat. My introduction to Dr. Daniels and the events that took place shortly thereafter were a defining and momentous time in my life. Recognizing that I was just as vain as the next person both humbled and excited me at the same time. And I was not the only one excited to hear her beauty secrets. The fact that we are genetically programmed to be concerned with our looks seemed like a natural door-opener in my mission to help educate people about health and nutrition. Our innate concern for our appearance is an inborn survival trait that programs us to listen to the health messages that our looks are sending us.

Our looks are a window to the state of our health. When we pay attention to our appearance and use natural means to improve our looks, those same natural methods improve our health.

Wrinkles, age spots, and acne are just early warning signals from our immune system. When our vanity motivates us to heed these signals with natural remedies, we are rewarded with beauty and improved health.

I immediately wanted to tap into this motivation in people. Instead of talking about the prevention of degenerative diseases as I have done for fifteen years, I suddenly had a burst of energy to talk and write about the body's restorative power to improve our physical appearance. Even when we become complacent or cynical about our appearance, deep inside we are still programmed to want to look and feel good. After all, it is our birthright.

But something has gone very, very wrong. More and more people are sick, suffering from one or many chronic conditions, and they don't look so good either. As Dr. Daniels says, our face reveals much about our state of health (see Table 6). Dr. Daniels made me fully aware that the beauty industry is just about as confusing an arena as the healthcare industry. It's hard to find truthful answers and practical solutions. There are plenty of people ready to have you spend hundreds or even thousands of dollars on lotions and potions, and even surgery, when the simplest solutions are at hand.

Table 1. The average cost of more "natural looking" treatments
(October 2008, Memphis, TN[1])

TREATMENT	COST
FACE LIFT	$4,000–$6,000
LASER "PEARL"	$1,800 1st treatment $1,200 additional treatments
BOTOX	
Frown wrinkles	$200–$400
Mild smile lines	$500–$700
Deep smile lines	$600–$1,200
MEDIUM-DEPTH CHEMICAL PEELS	$250–$500
COST FOR NEW FACE	$9,700–$13,100
(using scalpel, lasers, fillers, and chemicals)	

This book will show you quick, simple ways to reverse signs of aging—wrinkles, blemishes, gray hair, balding. You may never look eighteen again, and some of the ability to reverse the process will certainly depend on factors such as age and genetics. Still, your dedication to this program can take 10–20 years off your appearance. The huge side effect is that you'll feel great as well. Think about the far-reaching consequences of that for your family pictures, celebrations, and your ability to enjoy life without feeling self-conscious. Feeling inadequate and unattractive can diminish your enjoyment of life. Perhaps some of you have faced the frustration of spending thousands of dollars on beauty procedures only to find that the mark of time is still visible on your face, and that you've not only compromised your pocketbook, but your peace of mind as well. Never again!

I know Dr. Daniels' beauty secrets to be sound advice because even before I met her, I found that improved diet and hydration had made my wrinkles and gray hair disappear. I've also had the pleasure of trying out her remedies and seeing my complexion improve by the day. And I'm excited that even as years go by, I'm still able to keep wrinkles and gray hair at bay by using plants as medicine. Being seriously allergic to hair dyes, the natural solution to gray hair really got me excited. And it works!

And if you think it's too late for you to reverse the signs of aging, consider what my friend Dr. Paul Williams says: "It's true that you were never this old before, but you will also never be this young again either." In other words, there is always room for improvement.

So, let's get started!

Mitra Ray, Ph.D.

Dr. Mitra Ray received her Bachelor of Science from Cornell University, and her Ph.D. in Cell Biology from Stanford University Medical School. Her research has been funded by the National Institutes of Health and the American Cancer Society and published in prestigious journals. She is an author who is passionate about educating people on how to take control of their own health. She lectures around the world.

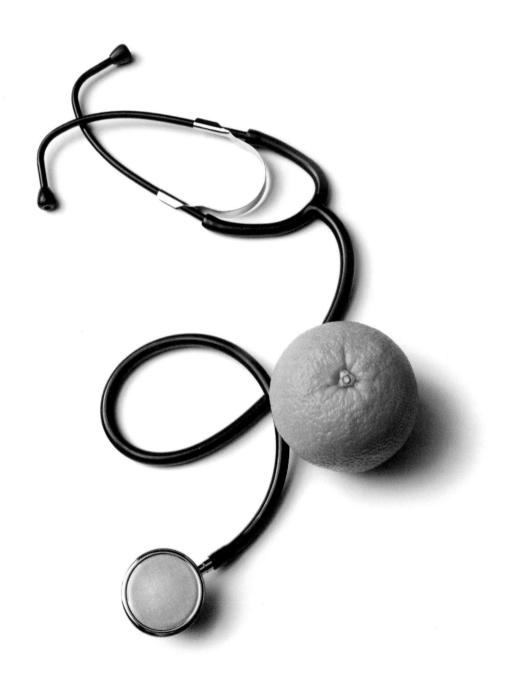

1.

Dr. Jennifer Daniels' Story

Dr. Jennifer Daniels never planned to become an expert on beauty and anti-aging, and her interest in this area came about almost accidentally. As a young girl of eleven, she met two sisters who were forty years old, yet looked like they were eighteen. She vowed to herself that she would look eighteen at the age of forty. As the years passed, she avoided foods that left her face looking older (you will learn which foods later in the book), got plenty of sleep, and checked the mirror a few times a year to make sure that she still looked healthy and youthful.

Like many young medical students, Dr. Daniels was on a tight budget. Because she'd grown up eating and preparing fresh produce, she tended to use her scant food dollars to buy things like potatoes and oranges in bulk, and she would live on these for weeks at a time. Generally, she could only afford to eat every other day. As she tells it:

"When I entered medical school, I seemed to stop aging for some reason, and actually started looking younger. At the time, I couldn't really put my finger on it. I was essentially fasting every other day! In retrospect, I realize

that this really gave my colon a chance to clean out and I wasn't holding on to any toxins, so my face was exceptionally clear and smooth. I finished medical school just thinking that my appearance was due to my genetics."

After medical school, Dr. Daniels worked as a physician on a Native American reservation, where she initially had a difficult time convincing members of that community to submit to a medical exam. It wasn't until a patient refused to be examined on the grounds that Dr. Daniels looked to be about the same age as his twelve-year-old daughter that she realized just how youthful she looked. Again, it seemed as though Mother Nature had dealt her a lucky hand, and she chalked her youthful looks up to good genes.

Eventually she chose to serve the inner city of Syracuse, N.Y., where she began what seemed to be a standard medical practice.

"I started prescribing drugs like every other doctor would, and I realized that my patients were not getting much better. I had recently decided to follow a vegetarian diet myself, and was feeling so healthy that I decided to suggest this lifestyle change to my patients as a way to improve their own health.

"I continued to educate myself about nutrition and herbs. I ultimately eliminated dairy, followed a whole food, plant-based diet, and began fasting regularly. Meanwhile, I noticed that those patients who were choosing to change their diet were not only healing their afflictions—their arthritis, their elevated blood pressure, their heart problems—but usually within about three weeks, they started looking years younger. This was very striking; so much so that after about two months, the patients were unrecognizable compared to when they first appeared in the office."

Within a few years, the word spread that Dr. Daniels' treatment made her patients look young and healthy, and people started coming in, some of them flying in from out of town, requesting that she treat them. They wanted to look young, healthy, and beautiful; they asked that Dr. Daniels help them look like her. Often these were patients with serious ailments that needed to be addressed, but they were far more concerned with how they looked—the diseases weren't what they wanted her help with. She explains:

"I had to get these patients to tell me exactly what it was that they wanted, because many of them were Caucasian women from the suburbs and I'm African-American. I would say, 'What do you mean look like me? How much of me do you want to look like?' And they would say, 'I'll take the skin color, too. I just want to look like you.' That is when I realized that something was up, that I was onto something."

And thus, her interest in how diet impacts beauty began. Being beautiful and looking youthful, she realized, had little to do with beauty products (because she didn't use any), and everything to do with eschewing the standard American diet. Processed food and animal products place a burden on the body that is too great to carry, and every aspect of health, including the appearance of the skin, suffers. She and her patients who followed the whole food, plant-based diet continued to feel healthy and youthful, and to maintain that glowing complexion that women desperately wanted her to help them achieve.

Over time, Dr. Daniels linked diet to every aspect of beauty and health. She says:

"Time marches on. Generally, I had a good complexion, but every now and then I would notice a wrinkle and say, 'Oh, my God! I have to get rid of this!'"

By experimenting with various healthy foods, cleansing practices, and fasting, she invariably found a way to get rid of the wrinkle, or age spot, or dry patch of skin.

What she shares with us in this book is how to reverse the signs of aging. Wrinkles, age spots, and blemishes are all the results of our lifestyle choices. The question that she answers for us is how to get rid of these *naturally*—without the use of chemicals, pills, or surgery. And it's important to point out that every "trick" you'll read about here is actually a wholesome and healthy way of living, part of a lifestyle that not only will keep you looking young, but will help you to be healthier than you've ever been before.

Dr. Jennifer Daniels received her undergraduate, pre-medical degree from Harvard University. She attended medical school at the University of Pennsylvania, where she simultaneously completed an MBA at the Wharton School of Business with a focus on healthcare management. Unlike most medical students, she was privy to an insider look at the business of healthcare. Within two years of prescribing pharmaceuticals, she quickly came to the conclusion that she was not upholding her promise as a physician to do what is best for her patients. She then took it upon herself to learn more natural alternatives for people. With her new holistic approach, she became so successful in making her patients look and feel better that word got out, and people began to fly in from around the country to see her. The Wall Street Journal did a feature story on her thriving practice within the inner city of Syracuse, N.Y.

Dr. Daniels had one young patient with type 2 diabetes who willingly chose the route of not taking insulin. Instead, he opted to modify his diet and lifestyle. He was thriving until he went on vacation and an alcohol binge sent him to the hospital. Although he was discharged from the hospital in good condition, this incident, along with Dr. Daniels' regular refusal to prescribe certain pharmaceuticals in her clinic, was fodder for The New York Office of Professional Medical Conduct (OPMC) to insist that she surrender all of her patients' medical records and her medical license. After years of futile litigation, along with discrimination from insurance companies, Dr. Daniels chose to shut down her clinic and retire from a formal medical practice.

Many articles have been written about Dr. Daniels' rough journey, but the saddest ones come from her own community, expressing their deep sense of loss at the closing of her practice.

Yet, Dr. Daniels' story continues to unfold into a brighter future, and we all stand to benefit from her new direction in life. Today she is committed to sharing her knowledge with a much wider audience, and benefiting more people than if she had remained in a standard medical practice. Her collaboration on this book exemplifies how she continues to reach out with her wisdom. In these pages she is able to keep her promise as a physician—to give you the knowledge that most serves you. And that's beautiful.

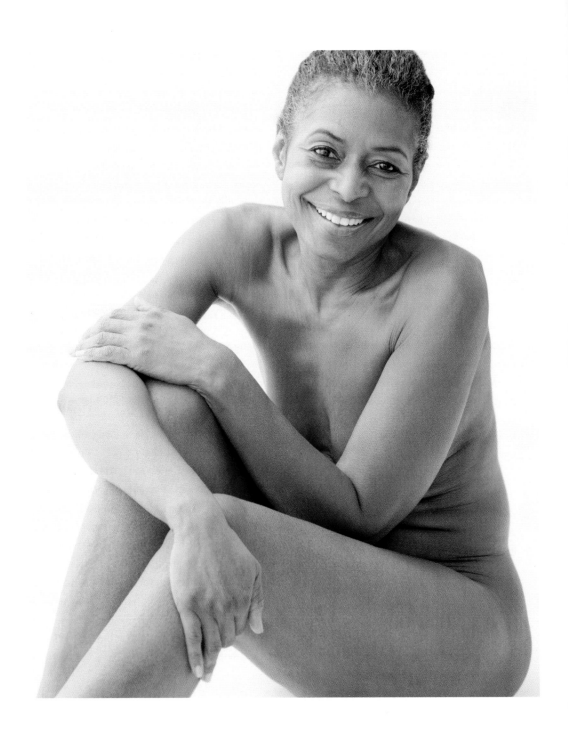

2.

How skin ages: theory and reality

We love to be pampered in the spa with a facial, massage, or sauna session. As a culture, we spend a lot of money on lotions and potions to have our skin feel and look better. We may even buy "clinically proven" cosmeceuticals—cosmetic products purported to have medical or drug-like benefits. In 2004, U.S. retail sales of cosmeceuticals accounted for over $12.4 billion. By 2010, the anti-aging market is expected to account for over $16.5 billion in sales.[2] These numbers do not even include the more expensive procedures such as laser resurfacing or cosmetic surgery. All in all, there is a great deal of money being spent in an attempt to recapture our youth.

The solutions in this book are easier on your wallet, and far better for your body. Furthermore, Dr. Daniels' medical background has allowed her to link bodily functions with beautiful skin in a way that is truly unique. While we will cite scientific literature where we can throughout the book, we wish to make a few important points about the suggestions herein. First, there is a great deal of controversy in the scientific literature as to the real cause of wrinkles, age spots, and other nuances of skin damage. Second, many of these beauty secrets are the brainchildren of Dr. Daniels. That is, these secrets came about over the years from Dr. Daniels' studying natural approaches to beauty and overall health, seeing what worked in her patients, and coming to intelligent conclusions about skin health, based on her knowledge of human physiology. Most importantly, what is outlined in this book works!

Our approach to beautiful skin is actually two-pronged: outside and inside the body. On the outside, Dr. Daniels' facial strips away—through microdermabrasion—dead cells and debris, and provides topical nutrients on the epidermal layer of the skin. And on the inside, since the body regenerates skin within a month, better diet and elimination help rebuild healthier skin. The effectiveness of the gut to absorb nutrition and eliminate toxins will drastically improve the quality of the new skin being made—hence the title of this book. With this two-pronged approach, you can expect to see results in a matter of days, and dramatic improvements over a month or two.

To understand the merit of the topical

approach, consider what most skin products aim to do. Whether you read brochures for a beauty product, a book on skin care, or even scientific literature, you will find that they all mostly focus on the second layer of the skin, the dermis. And within the dermis, the focus is on rebuilding collagen—it's the magic word you hear over and over again in the world of skin care. Why is collagen so important? Providing much of the skin's strength, collagen is one of the main building blocks of human skin. Dermal fibroblasts make precursor molecules called "procollagen," which is converted into collagen when the proper biochemical signals are triggered.

The reality is that the chemicals in creams and makeup do immediately affect the skin cells and accelerate aging. They can cause wrinkles and worsen existing wrinkles. Additionally, chemicals can even cause inflammation, redness, and blemishes.

Other than injecting chemicals into the dermal layer, most skin treatments are applied to the top layer, the epidermis. Research has shown that the topical application of a vitamin A derivative, retinoid, promotes the synthesis of collagen and reverses wrinkles.[3] This has proven effective for sun damaged skin, and it is expected that it may be effective in skin that is simply damaged as a result of aging. This is great news, because it means that the topical application of nutrients to the epidermis can penetrate to the dermis and be effective in reversing the signs of aging. This research supports many of the natural approaches in this book that involve applying nutrients directly to the face. On the other hand, most commercial creams don't contain nutrients that regenerate the skin. Instead, they contain chemicals foreign to the skin.

Why then do we as a society spend so much money on creams? We do so because they

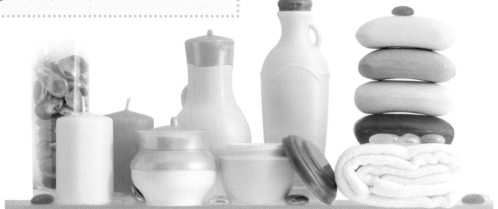

seem to work temporarily by trapping the moisture within the skin and plumping up the cells. So, for a few hours, your skin looks smooth. But there are hidden and immediate dangers to your skin from the use of chemicals. Many people unwittingly add insult to injury by putting on makeup over the cream. Just as medications used topically can have side effects throughout the body,[4] the reality is that the chemicals in creams and makeup *do* immediately affect the skin cells and accelerate aging. They can cause wrinkles and worsen existing wrinkles. Additionally, chemicals can even cause inflammation, redness, and blemishes.

There usually is no warning on skin care products and make up that they actually further damage the skin. For some, the use of makeup can damage the skin to the point that they are embarrassed to show their face in public without makeup. What we are recommending here is that you only use edible materials on your skin. If you bought a skin care product at the store that you wouldn't want to eat, then putting it on your skin is a counterproductive measure in the quest for youthful skin. You will absorb what you put on your skin just like you absorb food. The cream and the makeup simply paint a pretty face on top of skin cells that are aging and dying in the process. And if you do want to temporarily plump up your skin for an event, there is always Dr. Daniels' fabulous facial recommendation with edible products that

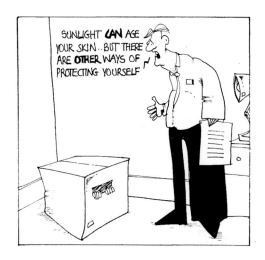

actually feed the skin with nutrients to help rebuild cells.

In reading about what causes wrinkles in the first place, much emphasis is put on sunlight damage. The prevailing theory on aging skin goes something like this: when skin is exposed to sunlight, UV radiation is absorbed by skin molecules that can generate harmful compounds, called "reactive oxygen species" (ROS) or, more commonly, "free radicals." These free radicals then cause oxidative damage to cellular components such as cell walls, lipid membranes, mitochondria, and DNA. This is called "oxidative stress." UV irradiation causes increased breakdown of collagen and decreased collagen formation. Free radical damage is thought to be the major cause of aging. The imperfect repair of this damage leads to what is called a "solar scar," manifesting as a visible wrinkle.

In other words, wrinkles are caused by a defective skin repair mechanism. This scientific name itself implies that sun damage causes wrinkles.

It is commonly believed that oxidative stress (caused by UV rays) is the major cause of wrinkles.[5] While it is true that UV damage may accelerate aging, the reality is that there is a constant turnover of cells in the body— old cells dying and new cells being rebuilt. In other words, it is the imperfect repair process that leads to persistent wrinkles. A robust repair process that could prevent wrinkles is dependent on proper nutrient building blocks. If the body does not get enough of the nutrients needed to build healthy new cells, wrinkles persist and worsen.

Besides wrinkles, there are many other types of skin damage. There is also new technology being developed every day to try to quantify each kind of skin damage or improvement. T. Wilhelm Callaghan and coworkers suggest that the effects of aging be defined by

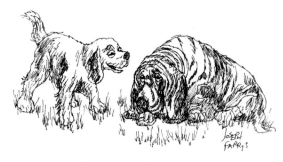

"Have you considered Botox?"

clinically observable key features such as skin roughness, surface texture, fine lines, wrinkles, skin color, and firmness.[6] We would like to focus on these measures of aging in this book since these are the features that are promptly improved by natural means.

Furthermore, an epidemiological study that was published in the *British Journal of Dermatology* indicates that age spots (senile lentigos, dyspigmentation) and wrinkles represent two different aging patterns.[7] In other words, there are separate and distinct causes of wrinkles and age spots. This is consistent with what Dr. Daniels has seen in her practice. And her approach to skin care emphasizes additional beauty practices that address the specific issues of age spots and wrinkles separately. She even addresses how to fine tune your beauty regimen in order to treat each type of wrinkle differently, and shows you how to focus on the particular blemishes and lines that concern you most.

In order to get the best benefit from this book, you should examine your skin using the measures mentioned above (skin roughness, surface texture, fine lines, wrinkles, skin color, and firmness) and rate your satisfaction with these areas. Take a picture and notice the difference in one week, two weeks, and one month. Beyond the first month, it is also a good idea to check your skin using these measures at least once a month. This allows you to catch and erase small issues easily, thereby maximizing your beauty benefits.

We actually recommend that you don't drive yourself crazy trying to address all of your wrinkles or blemishes at the same time with specific practices. Rather, focus on one or two issues at a time, and focus on hydration and diet for overall improvement.

Dr. Daniels has personally experienced all of the challenges addressed here, and reversed each by simple dietary changes or by applying edible materials to her skin.

So, how long can most people expect to be wrinkle and blemish free? Experiments have been done indicating that the life of a single cell can be extended indefinitely if proper nutrients are supplied and waste products are removed. In his book *Tissue Cleansing Through Bowel Management*, Bernard Jensen refers to the following study:

> Dr. Alexis Carrell at the Rockefeller Institute for Medical Research took small pieces of heart tissue from a chicken embryo to produce one of the most remarkable experiments in medical history. He attempted to demonstrate that under suitable conditions, the living cell could live a very long time, perhaps indefinitely.
>
> The heart tissue was immersed in a nutrient solution from which it obtained its food. Likewise, waste material was secreted into this same solution. Every day the solution was changed, taking away waste substances and providing fresh nutrients. It is amazing to report that this chicken heart tissue lived for 29 years in this fashion. It died one day when the assistant forgot to change the metabolized polluted fluid. In other words, autointoxication claimed this great masterpiece of experimental scientific investigation.[8]

Since this same principle of longevity applies to your skin cells as well, theoretically speaking, you can expect to look young as long as you cleanse your cells and provide the fresh nutrients regularly. It's a worthy cause that both of your authors are excited about. We also believe that if you look beautiful *on the outside*, it is because your organs are in excellent working order *on the inside*. Good health is the natural side effect of the practices within.

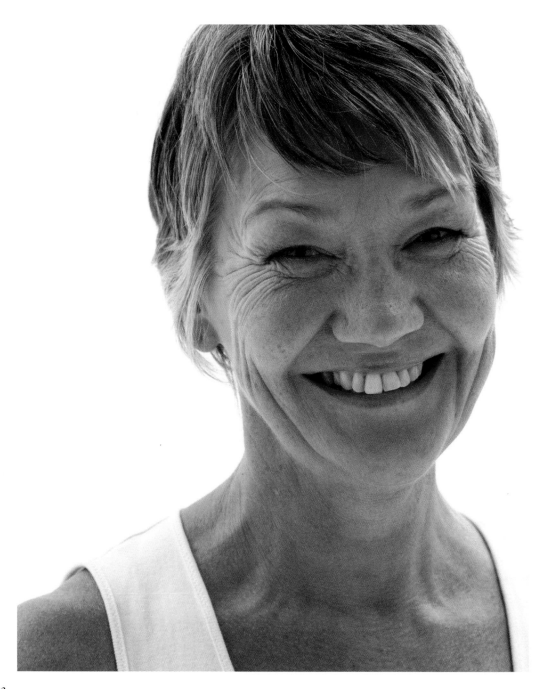

3

Erasing Blemishes and Wrinkles

How is it possible?

Imagine that you could literally erase blemishes and wrinkles. How would you feel if you looked in the mirror and started to see a younger you? How excited would you be if you showed up at parties and your friends commented on your youthful appearance and glowing skin? Can you get excited about that?

Some men take on a macho attitude, and refer to their wrinkles as "character lines" because they believe that wrinkles are permanent and nothing can be done about them. Not true! What we will talk about here is not an overnight solution—but neither do you have to wait months and months to get results.

The story of erasing blemishes and wrinkles begins within Dr. Daniels' medical practice.

After being frustrated with her patients' lack of healing from the use of pharmaceuticals, and being awakened at 2:00 A.M. with phone calls related to associated side effects of these drugs, Dr. Daniels began a very unique approach—she began offering her patients the choice to:

- do nothing,
- take drugs, or
- make diet and lifestyle changes, the most significant of which is to start eating a *whole food, plant-based beauty (WFPB) diet.*

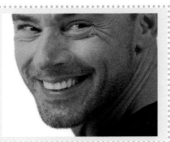

Some men take on a macho attitude, and refer to their wrinkles as "character lines" because they believe that wrinkles are permanent and nothing can be done about them. Not true!

Luckily, enough patients chose the path of most resistance—a change in diet—for Dr. Daniels to soon notice that people were not only healing themselves of their afflictions, but that she was no longer getting phone calls in the middle of the night. Her patients were sleeping through the night, and so was she. Also, her patients were looking better as they progressed on their WFPB diet.[a] There was a noticeable reduction of lines on the face, wrinkles, and blemishes. People were more confident, upbeat, and joyous about their appearance. Within two months of adopting a WFPB diet, they were unrecognizable compared to how they looked when they first walked into her practice. How satisfying for a physician to be able to offer health and good looks to her patients without needles, drugs, or surgery!

How did this change in her patients come about, and why are we interested? Well, we are interested because we want to look "beautiful." But what is beauty?

Beauty is when the cells in your body radiate a message of health to the world. This radiance is universally attractive. You feel good about yourself and others feel good about being around you. Beauty is an "inside job!"

And to discover how these changes in Dr. Daniels' patients came about, we'll need to explore the nature of skin and how it stays beautiful.

Beauty is when the cells in your body radiate a message of health to the world. This radiance is universally attractive. You feel good about yourself and others feel good about being around you. Beauty is an "inside job!"

---

[a] We advocate eating plants as much as you can. If you do choose to eat meat occasionally, be sure to read Appendix I about how to best neutralize the ill effects on your skin.

What is your skin?

Your skin reflects beauty and sensuality, and provides the sense of touch and pleasure. Covering 12–20 square feet of surface area, it is one of the largest organs in your body.[b] Your skin even shows emotions as you grow pale with fear or red with embarrassment. Your skin secretes pheromones which are odors that attract the opposite sex, and your pheromones can give another the sense of comfort and relaxation. Your skin provides protection from the environment. Your skin also helps to regulate body temperature either by using the contraction of fine muscles in the deep layers of the skin to retain heat—we've all had "goose bumps"—or by using sweat to cool.

We can enjoy all these important functions of the skin as long as it is nourished well and maintained properly. Since it is a living organ, the skin is nourished by food and damaged by toxins. These toxins include both the byproducts of normal biological activity, as well as chemicals that you ingest. Your skin is a reflection of how efficiently nutrients are being supplied to your entire body and how efficiently waste is being removed. Your skin is a reflection of what you are eating or not eating, and it is a reflection of waste prod-

---

[b] Since it is generally accepted that the skin is THE largest organ in your body, why are we saying that it is one of the largest? Well, size all depends on what we are measuring. For instance, if we consider surface area as a measurement, then the endothelium that lines our arteries and veins wins as the largest organ. Although individual endothelial cells are tiny in diameter (15 microns), because there are 10^{11} of them in the body, the surface area they cover can be 4,000–7,000 m^2 (about 6 tennis courts of surface area). Next is the surface area of the gut at 200 m^2, which exceeds that of the lungs (160 m^2) and the skin (<2 m^2) as an interface with the environment.

ucts that are retained in your body. You can get a reading on your internal organs from reading your face, as you'll soon learn. All told, your skin not only reflects your physical health, but it also reflects your emotional, mental, and spiritual states. This book will mostly focus on the physical component since this is easier to get a grip on intellectually, and it is easier to implement practically. Because the skin exfoliates and replaces itself about every twenty-seven days, beautiful skin can be obtained rather quickly with proper attention.

To begin to understand how to obtain beautiful skin, we need to understand more about the properties of the skin. We hear a lot in natural healing circles about how you should maintain an alkaline environment in the body.[c] While this is true of the blood, the skin is naturally acidic on the surface. One way your body maintains an internally alkaline environment is by displacing acid to the skin. The acid forms a waterproof protective barrier for the skin. As long as you eat what we call a whole food, plant-based beauty diet (WFPB diet),[d] the acid on the skin forms a beautiful, clear, protective layer called the "acid mantle."

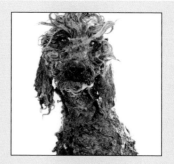

What is the significance of all of this? Well, most soaps are alkaline. Alkaline soaps overwhelm the skin and literally strip your protective acid mantle. This means that the moisture can now freely evaporate from your skin, allowing the skin cells to shrivel, and causing—you guessed it—wrinkles! So, "not using soap" is the number one step to keep your face from wrinkling.[e] You have to have a rule or discipline that you are NOT going to put soap on your face. This doesn't mean that you cannot cleanse your skin, only that you can't use soaps as cleansers. But not to fear! We'll tell you everything you need to know about how to cleanse and nourish your skin.

---

[c] The term pH is the "potential of hydrogen" and the pH scale ranges from 0 to 14, with 7 being neutral pH. Numbers below 7 are acidic and above 7 are alkaline. pH represents a logarithmic scale, which means that a pH of 9 is ten times more alkaline than a pH of 8. Normal skin pH ranges from the acidic range of 4.2 to 5.6, and varies throughout the body. Men generally have a lower pH (or more acidic skin) than women.

[d] See Chapter 4.

[e] For wrinkles, avoiding soap is even more important than diet. For age spots and acne, diet is the main key.

Additionally, much of your skin has hair follicles nurtured by sebaceous glands, which secrete a fatty substance called "sebum" (about 60% of which is triglycerides and free fatty acids). It is the combination of this oily sebum along with the acidic perspiration from your sweat glands that makes up the acid mantle. The acid mantle has several protective functions:

- It serves as a protective layer that prevents the growth of bacteria and fungi.

- It protects against the elements such as sun and wind.

- It helps to retain moisture and maintain a healthy, smooth glow.

- It makes your skin and hair waterproof!

So a key idea to understand is that your skin is naturally acidic. And this acid mantle protects your body from the elements and retains moisture.

What is a wrinkle?

In a perfect world, you have these perfect plump cells next to each other with no space between them (except an occasional pore), and the acid mantle on top. When light hits the surface of normal, healthy skin, it looks smooth and fabulous. The figures below are not meant to be highly technical; they have been simplified in order to show the function of the acid mantle on normal skin and the result of using soap.

When you use soap, the skin loses the acid mantle. The cells shrivel up due to dehydration, and don't line up nicely—similar to irregular teeth. When light hits the surface of dried-up skin, you see wrinkles. Sometimes there is a break, and this break will become a large pore. As we age, we will often see more wrinkles and large pores developing. Generally, dehydration is a big factor, secondary to soap use. This is why increasing water intake alone does not give dramatic relief

Figure 1. Normal, healthy skin

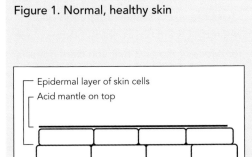

- Epidermal layer of skin cells
- Acid mantle on top

Figure 2. Dehydration
After use of soap or alkaline beauty products, wrinkles and pores are formed.

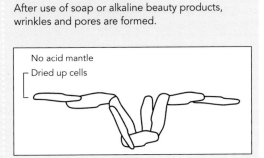

No acid mantle
- Dried up cells

from wrinkles. It is also necessary to stop water loss by restoring the waterproof layer. This holds water in the cells and stops new wrinkles from forming.

Deeper wrinkles and sags are caused by defects in the dermal layer of the skin. This is where the collagen that supports the skin is found. This collagen is especially sensitive to your nutritional status, and if you don't get enough phytonutrients (plant nutrients), such as vitamins, antioxidants, and minerals as well as essential fatty acids, you will lose that fullness and firmness of youthful skin, and deeper wrinkles will form over time. That is why the dietary changes are also necessary.

If you haven't appreciably changed your eating habits over the years, you may be wondering why you develop wrinkles and blemishes as you age. If you're more or less following the same diet that you did twenty years ago, you might wonder why your skin doesn't look like it did then. *The answer is that over time the intestines are less able to absorb nutrients as the result of twenty years of poor diet.* Those eating habits have changed your intestinal environment; and now, many nutrients are no longer being absorbed. This is going to be reflected in your face as wrinkles, age spots, or sagging skin since the nutrients necessary to maintain a beautiful face are not absorbed. Even the term "freckles," meant to sound cute, is really a reflection of toxins under the skin, visible to the eye by light filtering through the translucent epidermal layer. Genetically, we may have different amounts of pigmentation that allow some people to have more visible age spots, but in the end they are still age spots. There are limited studies that try to correlate ethnicity with aging skin, and the studies that have been done show conflicting results. So we cannot write them off simply as genetic traits. Age spots may also reflect common lifestyles within a group of people living in a particular region.[9] Never mind the genetics that determine the visibility of age spots; let's focus on the fact that age spots are caused by deposits of waste under the epidermis, and that they can diminish with cleansing practices.

Another misconception is that wrinkles just happen to show up as we age, and this un-truth is further validated by most of the literature on damaged skin. Yet, this supposition conflicts with the fact that new skin cells are being made daily even as we age. Our contention is that our physiology is not pre-programmed to change with age, but rather that a lifetime of poor eating habits changes our physiology. This is a key distinction—one whereby it is important not to blame yourself for habits of the past that you were not aware could hurt you. Rather see the bright side: *by reading this book you will have the knowledge and the power to build an improved, more beautiful complexion, despite your age. And your diet will be the most important habit that you will change.*

What is a blemish, or freckle, or age spot?

Underneath the first epidermal layer of skin cells is the blood supply; and when the body has lots of waste in the blood, it literally deposits the waste right under the top layers of skin cells (the epidermis). These are visible to the eye and these deposits are what we call "age spots," also called "freckles" or "blemishes."

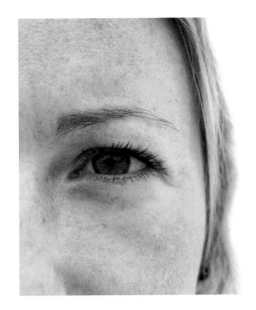

This dumping of trash under the epidermal layer can get out of hand. The body can deposit more and more and more waste products until lumps are formed, and it can even become a skin tag over time. Why is the body depositing these wastes in the skin? Because the organs involved in waste removal (liver, kidneys, lungs, and sweat glands) are overworked and undernourished, and waste deposits in the intestine are not being removed efficiently. And waste begins to accumulate in the blood. Eventually, this waste is deposited in an organ. When that organ is the skin, we call it an "age spot."

Figure 3. Age spot

(also called "freckles" or "blemishes")

Underneath the first epidermal layer of skin cells is the blood supply; and when the body has lots of waste in the blood, it literally deposits the waste right under the top layers of skin cells (the epidermis). These are visible to the eye and these deposits are what we call "age spots," also called "freckles" or "blemishes."

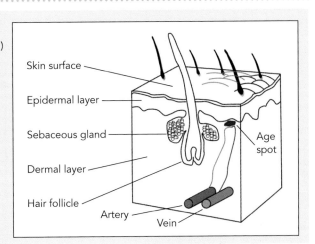

For instance, artificial sweeteners and preservatives, artificial flavors, and pesticides all challenge the liver. If the liver is no longer able to deal with the burden of these toxins, they remain in the blood. When the blood carries these toxins to your skin and deposits them there, they show up as an age spot. Because the waste is deposited right under your epidermal layer (see Figure 3), it becomes visible to the eye; and since this happens over time, we have come to call the resultant blemishes "age spots." We confuse time as the culprit, rather than the toxic chemicals that we have ingested over the course of many years. If you have numerous age spots and are really motivated to get rid of them, we want to let you know that it can be done via a "liver flush" that will take these spots and move them into the toilet.

An epidemiological study that was published in the *British Journal of Dermatology* indicates that age spots (senile lentigos, dyspigmentation) and wrinkles represent two different aging patterns.[10] In other words, there are separate and distinct causes of wrinkles and age spots. This finding is consistent with Dr. Daniels' experience. She has developed distinctly different beauty practices for erasing wrinkles, compared to those she recommends for erasing age spots. The fine tuning of beauty practices that work in different situations further bolsters the argument that what causes age spots is distinct from what causes wrinkles. We cannot simply write off all the nuances of skin problems as part of an ambiguous "aging process."

When the actual cause of acne is not treated and pills are used to trick the body into not putting waste into the skin, the waste goes to organs such as the kidney or brain; and this, in part, explains the serious and sometimes fatal side effects of popular acne therapies.

Figure 4. Normal sebaceous gland and hair follicle

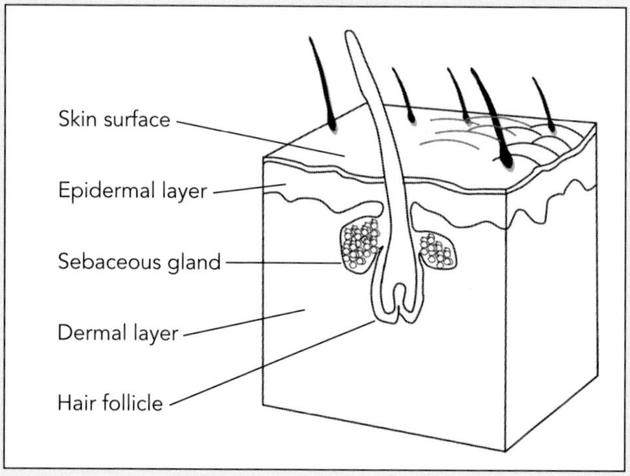

Skin surface

Epidermal layer

Sebaceous gland

Dermal layer

Hair follicle

What is acne?

Acne most often occurs in a young person with a diet rich in liquid toxins (e.g., sodas, dairy) and lacking in fiber (an inherent component of WFPB nutrition). Acne can also occur in an older person who mostly adheres to a WFPB diet, but also consumes alcohol or other liquid poisons. In both cases, the younger person and the person with a semi-decent diet both have a healthy enough blood cleansing mechanism that is anxious to get rid of the bacteria and wastes through the pores. If this material is allowed to circulate, it will harm vital organs. While acne may be unsightly, it is the body's way of protecting vital organs from harm. Cleverly, the body chooses to deposit these toxins and wastes in the sebaceous glands, which eventually become congested and clogged, expanding into a visible black head, white head, or cystic acne. It is important to treat the underlying cause of acne by removing these wastes from the blood or by not putting them into the blood in the first place. When the actual cause of acne is not treated and pills are used to trick the body into *not* putting waste into the skin, the waste goes to organs such as the kidney or brain; and this, in part, explains the serious and sometimes fatal side effects of popular acne therapies.[11]

The sebum excreted by the sebaceous glands is mostly composed of fatty acids and triglycerides. Acne is a reflection of bacteria, animal protein, and animal fat in the body. Generally, drinking milk will cause acne. Drinking soda pop will feed the bacteria and worsen acne. But acne does not spread from one part of the face to another, nor through person to person contact as some people may think. It is simply a heap of garbage from the blood that has been deposited in the sebaceous glands under the skin. Eat burgers, fries, coke, and ice cream, and you will get "zits." After a while, the toxins will seep out. Again, this doesn't mean acne will spread through contamination, but it will worsen if a person continues to eat foods that cause acne. People with sensitive skin can even get blemishes and irregular skin from canned and bottled foods.

Figure 5. Acne

A blackhead is an example of accumulated waste in the sebaceous gland.

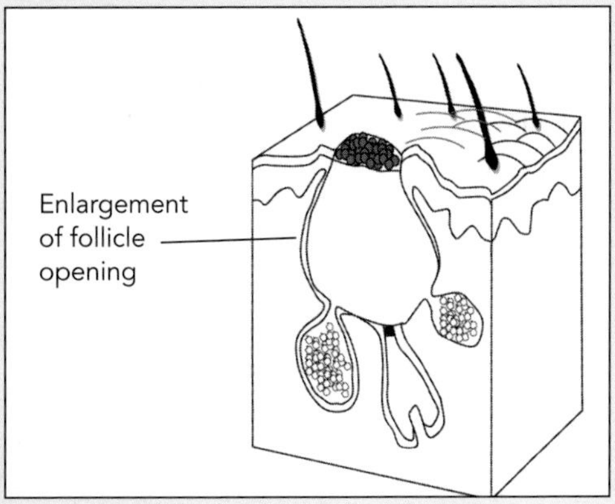

Enlargement of follicle opening

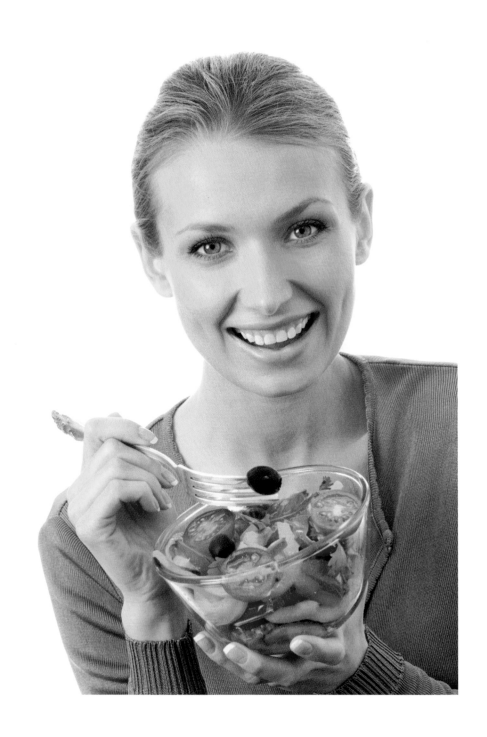

4.

Important Practices for Beautiful Skin: Diet

People who are in the business of skin care generally talk about lotions and potions. Yet, the most important aspect of beautiful skin is diet. When the diet is filled with foods that blemish and wrinkle the skin, it can add several years to your appearance, hours to your daily skin care routine, and hundreds of dollars to your beauty budget. With a skin-friendly diet, you can cut your skin care regimen to just a few minutes a day and look better, too.

Diet is the mainstay of beautiful skin, and it is when people have an unhealthy diet that they feel the need to spend thousands of dollars to visit the plastic surgeon and the skin care section at the cosmetics counter.

Eating Organic

The foods that you eat should be 100% organic. Be fastidious about this! Depending on your will power, you may have to go to a health food store that sells all organic to purchase your produce; when you see conventionally grown food, which often costs considerably less than organic produce, you may be tempted to buy the cheaper, non-organic product. Dr. Daniels has a rule that if it's not organic, it doesn't enter the house! All those pesticides get stored in age spots, and they are very difficult for your liver to filter out. In general, organic produce has 1/3 of the pesticides that regular produce has—so you still get some of those residues even when you eat organic. And if you eat non-organic, those chemicals can overwhelm your immune system and liver, thus giving you all sorts of health and cosmetic challenges that you don't need. Such chemicals often are not removed by the liver, kidneys, or lungs, and get deposited in the skin causing age spots or acne. Even if the immune system does remove these chemicals from the circulation, the increased demand of nutrients required for this task leaves the skin short changed, and wrinkles are the result.

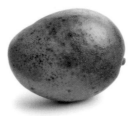

The Green Drink

Yuck! Green Drink? Are you kidding? That doesn't sound good at all!

Well, you can relax because the recipe we offer is actually quite easy on the taste buds, and after a week you will come to love it. It's basically a fruit smoothie with some dark leafy greens thrown in for beauty's sake. Remember that you are on your way to a more beautiful you. Not only will the Green Drink make your skin glow, but it will also give you far superior energy compared to the typical morning ritual of coffee or tea.

Start your day with a Green Drink. You will notice the difference in two days; your friends will notice the difference in four days! Barley Green types of additives will not have the same effect.

Dark leafy greens have a very high dose of nutrients that can give you the results you are looking for—a reversal of previous damage to your skin. Hence, the name we are using to emphasize the point—the Green Drink! The fruits in the Green Drink act more as sweeteners, but remember: buy organic. The organic fruits also provide the skin with phytonutrients that will help to neutralize free radicals that can otherwise damage your collagen and make you look older. The flax seeds support collagen formation and reduce sags.

The Green Drink is phenomenal because it not only gets rid of wrinkles, but also gets rid of the big sags under the eyes.

For making larger quantities with more greens, or to make enough for a whole family, a Vitamix® is a great tool, and worth the investment. It makes it a breeze to make a Green Drink with a smooth texture. You can play with various dark leafy greens. There are many varieties of kale. Additionally, try Swiss chard, bok choy, collard greens, mustard, turnip, beet greens, carrot greens, spinach, or parsley.

Make the drink a thinner consistency if you tend toward constipation, and make it a thicker consistency if you tend toward diarrhea.

Once you get going on this, it will occur to you that the Green Drink is also useful for using up whatever fresh produce you might have in your fridge or fruit basket that is too ripe to enjoy. Just toss it into the blender instead of throwing it into the trash! Also, the parts of veggies that no one wants to eat, like the stems of broccoli—you guessed it—

go in the Green Drink. More fiber, better bowel movements, better skin!

For added variety and even more savory Green Drink possibilities, find a copy of *Green for Life* by Victoria Boutenko (Raw Family Publishing, 2005). The book also features testimonials from people who had serious health challenges before learning about the power of leafy greens, and some of the health benefits they describe include skin improvement.

"My liver spots have faded noticeably."

"I was born with eczema and I had to take heavy medications all my life. . . .This remarkable beverage not only greatly improved my skin condition, but I am also sleeping much better—without scratching."

Dr. Daniel's simple STARTER recipe for one person:

3 large kale leaves, chopped
2 bananas – very ripe, frozen or fresh
1 fleshy fruit chopped, frozen or fresh
1/4 cup flax seeds or chia seeds
1 tsp. milk thistle
Enough water to make 6 to 8 cups

Put flax and milk thistle in blender. Blend until powder-like. Add other solid ingredients and 3 cups of water. Blend until liquefied. Add more water to make 6 to 8 cups, and blend. Drink throughout the day. Using some frozen fruit will help to make the Green Drink a little cooler, and this helps with the strong taste of the greens. Dr. Ray also likes to use organic, red, seedless grapes to sweeten and cool the drink. You can pluck them off the stems and freeze them in large quantities so they are ready to use.

Whole food, plant-based beauty diet

It is important to eat a whole food, plant-based beauty (WFPB) diet. Because animals are higher on the food chain than plants, toxic chemicals such as herbicides and pesticides get super-concentrated in the fatty tissue of animals. Plants have less fat and far fewer toxins. In their whole food form, they have a tremendous amount of fiber, which acts as a sponge once it enters the body and sequesters toxins, keeping them from getting into your skin. Animal flesh has no fiber and super-concentrated toxins. The immune system, when challenged with animal products, simply does its job of protecting your vital organs by depositing these toxins in your skin. These toxins can show up as age spots and steal your good looks from you.

You also want to eat whole foods because *processed foods drain your body of water and enzymes*—so even a vegan pizza, because it is processed, will take a whole lot of water to process, and your body will have to produce many enzymes to digest it. Digestion is a tremendous amount of work for the body, and it goes through the effort simply to gain some vital nutrients. Giving the body any kind of processed food reduces the efficiency of the whole system, and this extra work for little benefit has serious consequences for the skin. The water, energy, and the body's resources (such as amino acids) needed to make those enzymes could be directed toward keeping your skin wrinkle-free and blemish-free, rather than processing the pizza you just ate. So whenever you eat processed food, you are sacrificing your beauty.

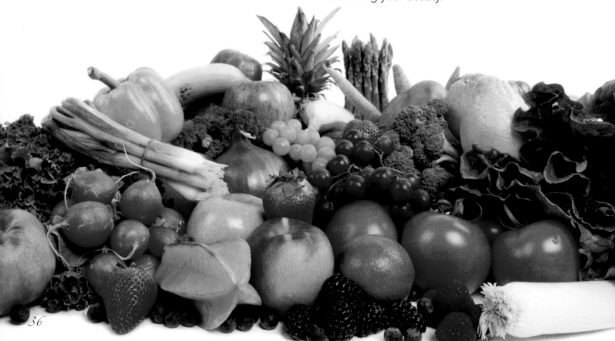

Table 2. Foods that promote beauty and health

	DESIRABLE PREPARATIONS	UNDESIRABLE PREPARATIONS
ORGANIC FRUITS	Raw, frozen Fresh juices, smoothies, and poached fruit	Dehydrated Packaged with preservatives such as sulphur, herbicides, pesticides, and added sugar Canned
ORGANIC VEGETABLES	Raw Fresh juices or smoothies Made into soups (no oil or fat) Grilled (without oil) Steamed Boiled Frozen	Dehydrated Packaged with herbicides, pesticides, added sugar, and preservatives such as sulphur Avoid cooking with oil, butter, or any other fat Microwaved Canned
ORGANIC BEANS AND LEGUMES	Soaked overnight and simmered on stove Prepared in slow cooker Prepared in pressure cooker Sprouted	Avoid instant foods that require only heating and/or adding water Canned beans are not good for facial beauty
WILD OR ORGANIC WHOLE GRAINS (preferably gluten-free, such as wild rice, brown rice, and teff)	Cooked as per directions – usually stove top preparation with water Rinsed, soaked or sprouted	Avoid pre-made foods that require only heating and/or adding water Avoid gluten if you have puffy eyes or crow's feet
ORGANIC SEEDS (flax seeds are best)	Raw Ground up right before use Soaked overnight (¼ cup whole flax seed + 1 cup water) for maximum essential fats absorption. Stir in the morning and drink.	Made into oils
ORGANIC NUTS	Raw with limited intake – a fistful maximum; best consumed as a condiment	Roasted, with or without salt With preservatives and additives Stale As a nut butter with added salt and other chemicals

Table 3. Ingested substances that detract from beauty and health

1. SOCIAL POISONS—tobacco, alcohol, coffee, and black tea.

2. OVER-THE-COUNTER MEDICATIONS—pain killers, laxatives, antihistamines, sleeping pills, cold and flu remedies—are all perceived as chemicals by your body and thus contribute to age spots, wrinkles, and acne.

3. ALL ANIMAL PRODUCTS (unless specifically included in a diet individually prescribed to you by a qualified health professional). These include cheese, butter, and other dairy; eggs; meat, fish, fowl, and even wild game.

4. ALL BEVERAGES EXCEPT GOOD, CLEAN WATER—no sodas, no funny "health" drinks made from "natural" ingredients.

5. CHEWING GUMS AND BREATH MINTS—especially sugarless ones.

6. PACKAGED FOODS—with or without chemical additives that you cannot pronounce.

7. OILS—olive oil, "cold-processed" oils, fish oils, margarine, and fried foods. Take flax seed as described in Table 2 to meet your body's essential fat needs. In 90 days, you will stop craving oily, fatty foods.

8. HIGH PROTEIN POWDERS, AND BARLEY-GREEN TYPE PRE-MADE DRINKS. These are overly concentrated and pull water from your system for digestion. This creates relative dehydration, resulting in wrinkles and sag lines.

9. AMINO ACID SUPPLEMENTS, ISOLATED VITAMIN SUPPLEMENTS—anything that is not made from whole food and is not backed up by independent clinical trials on the product itself.

Just to be clear, lets really explore what we mean by a whole food, plant-based beauty diet. "Vegetarian" and "vegan" are names we use for people who avoid certain foods; we love to label objects, people, places. In reality, everyone makes choices that are based on different motivations, and each of us eats quite uniquely. The terms "vegetarian" or "vegan" can refer to dietary habits that harm your looks, or they can refer to dietary habits that improve your looks. Not all vegetarians and vegans follow a whole food, plant-based beauty diet. Avoiding animal products isn't enough to ensure true health and beauty.

So, in trying to communicate the diet we are recommending, we want to be certain that our readers are fully aware of what foods will create the beautiful results they seek and what foods will detract from their good looks.

In other words, *it is the consumption of particular foods, rather than a particular diet, that is important for beauty.* It is a diet rich in plants in their whole food form, which particularly enhances beautiful skin. In addition, we want to clarify certain methods of preparation that are wholesome, and those that are not. Buy organic and/or locally grown. You can use most vegan cookbooks, but simply avoid the oil and other beauty-detracting ingredients found in many of the recipes.

Going out to eat

Being social—which usually involves food—fills the heart. So what to do when you go out in a world full of choices that don't serve your beauty? First of all, commit 100% to a WFPB diet at home. Over time, this simple commitment will make it easier and easier to make good choices when you go out. You will natu-

Table 4. Sources of oxidative stress (free radical production)

CIGARETTE SMOKE (EVEN 2ND-HAND SMOKE)	ALCOHOL	ANIMAL PRODUCTS
STRESS	RADIOACTIVITY	OIL SUPPLEMENTS
SMOKED, GRILLED, PRESERVED FOOD	PHARMACEUTICALS	UV RAYS
COOKED FATS	OZONE	POLLUTED WATER
NORMAL METABOLISM	SMOG	EXERCISE
	PHASE I ENZYME BYPRODUCTS	MICROBIAL INFECTION

rally adapt. You will find ways of avoiding certain foods, and enjoying the company instead. If you have the choice, fill up on homemade food before you go. That way even if you do choose to eat foods that deter from your beauty, you will eat less of them. Also, stay well hydrated. In Chapter Six, we will discuss why cleansing practices may be beneficial as well.

Appropriate Supplementation

Along with eating a variety of plants and making sure to get those dark leafy greens in your diet, you can additionally boost your plant nutrient variety with whole food based supplementation, flax seeds, and additional minerals. One brand of whole food based supplementation has been clinically shown to increase key nutrients in the blood, reduce oxidative stress, and improve circulation.[f] This is good news for the skin. Because of these clinical results, both Drs. Ray and Daniels use this supplement personally. A broad base of bioavailable micronutrients has been shown to improve skin hydration, skin elasticity and roughness, and capillary blood flow. All of these improvements translate to visible changes that can be noticed within a few months.

Lets discuss "oxidative stress" and how it damages the skin. Underneath the epidermis is the dermis, where important components of the skin—such as blood capillaries, hair follicles, sweat glands, nerve endings, and oil glands—are embedded in a matrix of collagen, elastic tissue, and reticular fibers. Sagging skin and deep wrinkles can occur when there is a breakdown in the structural components of the dermal layer from free radical damage. The integrity of the dermal layer is important for structural as well as functional reasons.

Free radicals are the normal byproduct when our cells are burning glucose to create the energy currency of the body, adenosine triphosphate (ATP). Free radicals can cause damage because they are missing an electron and they try to steal electrons randomly from stable molecules in the body. In addition to normal metabolism, we experience a wide variety of other sources of free radicals (see Table 4).

Free radicals are implicated in causing premature aging and disease in the body. A wide variety of antioxidants from plant sources can neutralize these free radicals before they can attack our cellular components; and, in so doing, can help to prevent aging at the molecular level.

In the dermis, free radical damage causes wrinkles by activating enzymes that break down collagen. You will notice wrinkle lines,

---

[f] Juice Plus+® is a whole food based nutritional supplement that has a broad base of plant nutrients and has clinical research to prove efficacy. (www.juiceplus.com)

especially around the lips of a smoker. Also, sun worshippers often have wrinkled skin from too much sun. A diet rich in processed food and animal products can cause similar damage. Smokers and sun worshippers, as well as the rest of us, can improve the health of the skin through whole food based supplementation because research has shown that whole food based supplementation can increase the amount and variety of antioxidants circulating in the blood.

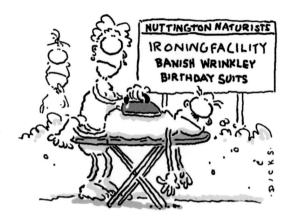

Another good tip is to include flax seeds in your diet, regardless of what else you're eating. The essential fatty acids in flax seeds that are freshly ground up and mixed with water help to rebuild collagen. This is one other way in which the Green Drink is a miracle for the body and skin. It's the perfect medium for flax seeds, since it automatically provides enough liquid to hydrate the freshly ground seeds, and the flavors of the ingredients all work well together.

Regular detoxification is essential to beauty, and helping the liver to better do its job of filtering out toxins will improve the quality of the blood going to the skin. When food is digested, the nutrients and toxins are absorbed by the intestines and enter the blood supply via the portal vein, which first sends the blood to the liver before circulating that blood to the body. The liver has many key functions, one of them being to remove toxins in the blood before the blood circulates to other organs. The

liver does this through the activation of phase I and phase II detoxification enzymes that tag and remove waste from the blood. Some of this waste is further processed by the kidneys, and then excreted through the urine; and some enters the bile and gallbladder, and is then emptied into the intestines. From here, the final step occurs when the bowels empty and waste leaves the body. Also, phase I enzymes can actually increase the free-radical load unless neutralized by plant antioxidants. It is especially important to note here that phase II enzymes don't even get activated until enough key plant nutrients are found in the diet.[13] Taking whole food based supplementation from a variety of plants can improve the liver's ability to supply cleaner blood to the body, which is the key to health and, hence, to beauty.

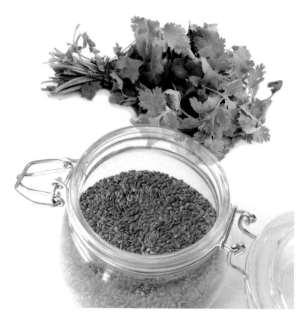

In fact, the whole system of detoxification depends on plant nutrients in order to work efficiently. For instance, plants such as cilantro, along with proper hydration, can keep the kidneys in good working order; but should the kidneys fail to remove waste properly, the sweat glands come into play and remove excess waste through the skin. This will increase body odor. While your blemishes may not indicate total organ failure, they do indicate an organ slowdown in the removal of waste from your blood. The cosmetic defects (acne, blemishes, and wrinkles) are just a gentle warning.

Regular Fasting

If you want a super gorgeous complexion, Dr. Daniels says:

"It is impossible to maintain beautiful skin on three meals a day!"

If you regularly have only two meals a day and stop eating by the afternoon, then your body has many hours to process that meal, to detoxify—to tag and remove those chemicals in an orderly fashion through your liver, your colon, your kidneys, and your lungs—so that nothing is left over in the blood to form a wrinkle or a blemish. For instance, if you sip on a Green Drink all morning, and then have a simple meal of vegetables with brown rice or lentils in the afternoon, then you will feel quite satisfied, and may not feel the need to eat later in the day. This will allow for a good night's rest and skin regeneration.

Fasting speeds up the detoxification process. Actually, "detoxification" is a term that you'll hear, but we prefer to think of it as "rejuvenation."

If it were up to us, we would redo the jargon in the literature and call the whole thing the process of rejuvenation. "Detoxification" doesn't sound nice. It is the natural design of the body to heal itself, "to rejuvenate."

How often should you fast? Dr. Daniels says:

"Hey, if you want those good looks, fasting once a week is what I consider a very good habit. It allows your body to catch up and fully digest the food, and clean out toxins, and turn back the hands of time."

Is it safe for anyone to fast? As long as your body mass index BMI is over 23 and you are currently not taking medications, it is perfectly safe to fast once a week.[9] Again, the medical establishment may not agree with this. Still, we can look to so many old traditions from different parts of the world and see that fasting has been a time-honored practice in many cultures. Furthermore, our physiology has adapted to fasting because of our history on this planet where starvation, until recent times, has been the number one challenge for the survival of our species. Even for wild animals today, the number one threat is food scarcity. We have adapted to using periods of food scarcity as a time to heal the body. This important process of healing and repair has been all but lost in modern times. Self-imposed food scarcity is known as "fasting," and the payoff is that it allows the body to heal rather quickly. Most species have physiological adaptation methods to survive periods of food scarcity. Here, we are only discussing one day a week. Still, please make sure you do the simple calculation of your BMI and make sure it is greater than 23. If your BMI is less than 23, or you are under 18 years of age, or if you have any medical conditions, we recommend only medically-monitored fasting (see Resources).

Drink plenty of water on the day that you fast.

$$\text{Your BMI} \ (kg/m^2) = \frac{(\text{Your weight in pounds} \times 703)}{(\text{Your height in inches})^2}$$

[9] To calculate your body mass index (BMI), you can either use the formula given if you are good at such calculations, or go to the Internet and find a BMI calculator where you can plug in your weight and height.

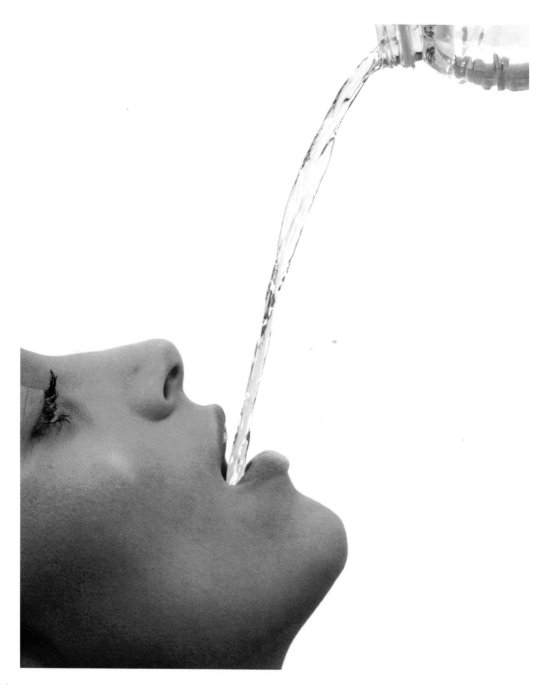

5.

Important Practices for Beautiful Skin: Hydration

Your body is 72% water. You can imagine that even the slightest dehydration can be detrimental to how your body works, and this will be reflected in how you look. Water makes up most of the blood that circulates nutrients to the body, and it makes up most of the milieu inside the cell that allows for chemical reactions to take place. Water also flushes out toxic chemicals and metabolic wastes from the body. When water is in short supply, the immune system shortchanges non-critical tissues such as the skin. In other words, dehydration of 5% may cause the immune system to reduce blood flow to the skin by 20% in order to allow the brain or the kidneys to maintain 100% blood flow. Over time, this causes wrinkles and sags.

So how much water do you need to drink? Consider that beauty is attained through a daily cleansing of the body. You need to drink enough water to urinate at least 3-4 times a day! The advice is to start your day with a glass of water and continue throughout the day to drink water 10 minutes prior to meals or in between meals. Before going to bed, have a glass of water ready (covered) by your bedside so that you can have that first glass in the morning, before your feet hit the ground. If you have a job or occupation where you don't have the time to go to the bathroom in the daytime, then begin drinking as soon as you get home. If water drinking extends to bedtime, this may mean getting up several times during the night so that you can be beautiful during the day.

Understanding Drinking Water

Besides hydration, water also can provide us with minerals. At least, that was the original plan. Industry has polluted all of the water on the planet. Any attempt to clean up this water still leaves it short of perfect. Yet we want clean water, with the minerals, and without the pollutants. Proper hydration and mineral intake are key components of your beauty regimen.

Since many people are confused by the choices of different types of water, we will discuss the pros and cons of these less-than-perfect choices. We won't discuss more complicated concepts such as ionized water and clustered water. The reason for this is that most people will not use them for a beauty regimen that requires such large volumes of water consumption, for both drinking and cooking. That leaves us with six basic choices for water, and all have their benefits and disadvantages:

- distilled water

- mineral water

- spring water

- reverse osmosis water

- alkaline water

- tap water, processed through a carbon filter

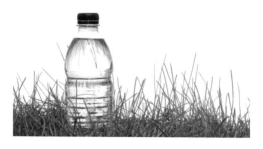

Distilled Water

Let's start with why the medical establishment is dead against distilled water. It is acidic and aggressive. After 3-4 years of drinking distilled water you will get osteoporosis, cavities, and weakened blood vessels. So why would we be so crazy as to recommend it? It is that old theory of healing – often that which can kill you can also heal you if used prudently.

How is distilled water made? Water is first boiled and the resulting steam is then condensed and filtered. Purified water molecules are chemically aggressive by nature because they hate to be alone. It is the very aggressive nature of distilled water that can mobilize

Table 5. Approximate water intake for beauty and health

Weight	Water intake (quarts)	Water intake (ounces)	Water intake (liters)
100–120	2+	64+	1.9+
120–180	3+	96+	2.8+
180–240	4+	128+	3.8+
240–300	5+	160+	4.7+

toxins in the body just as it mobilizes minerals out of the body. As one example of distilled water's real healing properties, Dr. Daniels has found that it can even mobilize encrusted waste from the joints of arthritic patients. You can also lower the acidity with a squeeze of fresh lemon, although this is not necessary on a WFBP diet. That's because if you really stick to a WFPB diet and do your Green Drink, you will be able to neutralize the acidity from the water. And as for the loss of minerals from the body, fortunately we can replenish the minerals for the month or so you are focusing on your beauty regimen, or whenever you choose to drink distilled water. Also remember, you have to drink distilled water without any minerals for many years to develop osteoporosis or cavities. If you already have weakened bones or are worried about mineral loss, just add more mineral supplementation as recommended below.

There are three basic types of *liquid mineral supplements* that will work:

- trace minerals

- plant-derived minerals (chelated to plant peptides)

- colloidal minerals

Use brands that have at least 30 minerals, and those with 78 are best. Take about 2 tablespoons per day; for those who have less bone density, take ¼ to ½ cup daily.

If you suspect that you have weakened bones, simply test yourself by putting pressure on your wrists, such as in a partial push up. If your wrists feel weak and unstable, this is an indication of loss of bone density.

Mineral Water

Mineral water is found in beautiful mountains where the water flows through earth that has a high density of crystallized minerals, such as

An adequate amount of water intake is 1+ quart per 60–70 pounds of your weight per day.

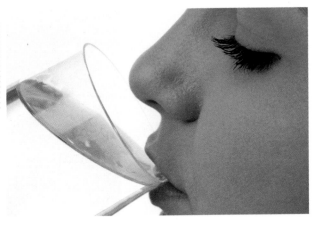

calcium crystals. Unfortunately, mineral water can also have inorganic forms of minerals that are unusable by the body, so they end up as encrusted waste. Thus, the regular use of mineral water can lead to arthritis and bone spurs.

The real healing power of mineral water is when you jump in a mineral water stream. Bathing in mineral water from these mountains pulls toxins out of the body. A word of caution about spas that tout mineral baths – usually they are diluting the mineral water with 50-75% tap water and then the healing quality is lost in dilution.

Spring Water

This is simply water before it goes to a treatment plant. On our planet, at this time, unfortunately this means that it has trace amounts of dioxins, heavy metals, PCBs, pesticides, pharmaceutical and other chemical waste, and even sporadic parasites. At one time, during the pre-industrial era, spring water would have been great to drink as it is mineralized with composted plants, which is the ideal source of minerals. Alas, the pollutants.

Reverse Osmosis Water

Reverse osmosis water is very similar to distilled water in that it is aggressive and acidic, but otherwise very clean water. With the addition of liquid minerals, reverse osmosis water is a relatively economical and long term, practical solution. You can buy an appliance for making reverse osmosis water in the home. This option is less expensive than installing distillation equipment and more convenient than buying bottled distilled water all the time.

Alkaline Water

The concept of drinking alkaline water comes about as a way of compensating for a diet rich in processed food and animal products,

The real healing power of mineral water is when you jump in a mineral water stream. Bathing in mineral water pulls toxins out of the body. Spas that tout mineral baths are usually diluting the mineral water, allowing the healing quality to be lost in dilution.

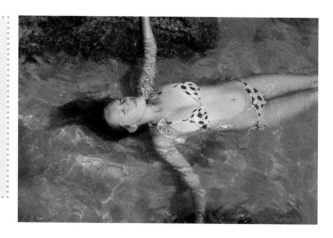

all of which overwhelm the body's own ability to regulate the delicate acid/alkaline balance. Remember how the body maintains an internal alkaline environment and has an external acid mantle for protection. And this balance can be perfectly maintained on a WFPB diet. Now if you are not on a WFPB diet, then drinking alkaline water may initially make you feel great for about 3-4 days, which gets people excited. But it will not bring you more beauty.

This is because there are two ways to alkalinize water: alkaline drops, or water that gets split into acidic and alkaline water by an appliance you can purchase. With the alkaline drops, you are just changing the pH of the polluted water. This change in pH may be appreciated by the body's enzymatic machinery for a few days, but eventually the toxins in the water and diet will put things back to status quo. And when water is split, the alkaline toxins come with the alkaline water.

Tap Water Processed through a Carbon Filter

This method is simply not sophisticated enough to match the new plethora of pollutants in our water.

In conclusion, we recommend that the best long term solution is to invest in either a home-distillation unit or a reverse-osmosis filter. Add liquid minerals as often as possible, and as directed previously in this chapter.

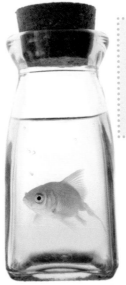

Industry has polluted all of the water on the planet. Any attempt to clean up this water still leaves it short of perfect.

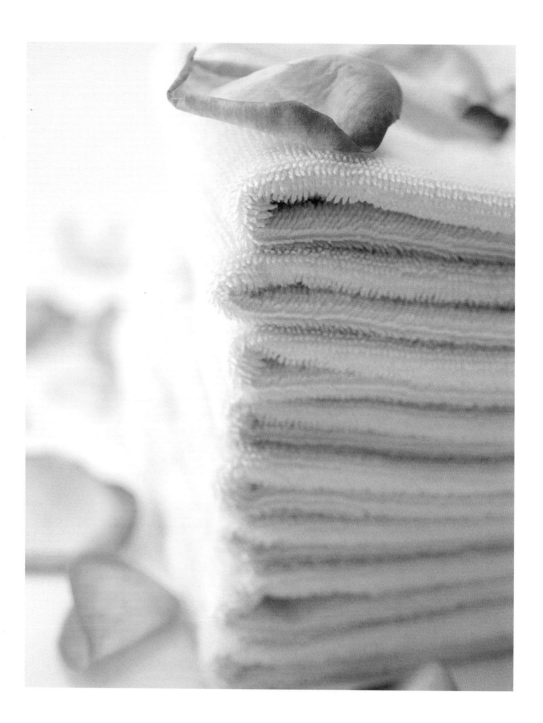

6

Important Practices for Beautiful Skin: Enemas

Appreciating the Power of Enemas

Why should we do enemas? Because enemas are highly effective at getting rid of age spots and wrinkles. In the beginning, if you follow our recommended procedure, you can do them once or twice a day until your face is clear. An enema provides deep cleaning. It cleans out the colon so that more toxins can be brought from the blood to the colon for cleaning. Putting more effort into your diet means that fewer enemas will be needed over time in order to reach your desired goal.

Be aggressive about getting toxins out of your body. For men, generally having three bowel movements a day works; women should have more. This is because all that most guys want is a reasonably clear face: a nice, rugged, masculine look will usually work for them. But most women really want satiny smooth skin with no age spots, and for that they have to go the extra step of doing enemas. The enemas Dr. Daniels recommends are very gentle. Initially, doing enemas daily will be critical in order to get rid of age spots.

Once you are satisfied with how clear your skin is, you can taper down to between one and four enemas a month to maintain your good looks. If you space your enemas as far apart as once a month, often new blemishes will appear. Your time investment is minimal—15 minutes if you do it quickly, or 30 if you take your time—and your reward is clear skin. Colonics are NOT necessary but some people may prefer them. If you do an enema in the evening, you will look great in the morning! If you want to look great in the evening, do it in the morning.

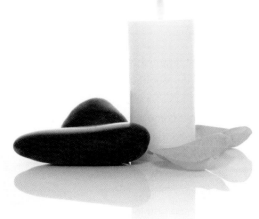

Dr. Daniels' Gentle Enema Procedure

MATERIALS NEEDED:

- 1 "OLD STYLE" ENEMA BAG—RINSE BEFORE FIRST USE

- 1 FULL-SIZE TOWEL

- 1 QUART MEASURE

- 1 THERMOMETER

First, fill quart measure with 2½ cups of room temperature distilled water. Add near boiling distilled water to make one quart. Stir to evenly distribute the heat. The final temperature should be 105 degrees or so. You can double-check this with a thermometer the first time to make sure that the water is not too hot. It should feel pleasantly warm when you wiggle your finger in it. Warm water enemas will improve your appearance more quickly than those done at room temperature.

*Note of caution: Each time you do this, test the temperature of the water coming **out of the insertion tube** with your fingers to make sure that the water entering your body is not too warm.*

The first time that you use your enema bag, rinse it thoroughly, and assemble your bag, tubing, stopper and nozzle as per the instructions that come with the kit. You can find suggestions for purchase and use of equipment at http://www.enemabag.com/how_to_take_an_enema.html. We are recommending that you take a simple, 1 quart, warm water enema and nothing more elaborate.

Note: **You must be well-hydrated before you start the enema. Drink at least a quart of water.**

1. Spread the towel on the floor in your bathroom near your toilet.

2. Make sure stopper for the flow is off and pour prepared water into enema bag.

3. Hang enema bag on a towel bar or hook and within reach of where you will be lying down.

4. Allow water to flow into tubing and then stop the flow once water has reached the nozzle and you are satisfied that it is not too hot.

5. Lie on your left side. Take a few deep breaths to make sure you are relaxed.

6. Make sure stopper is closed and in your hand so you can control the flow of water once you begin.

7. Insert nozzle into your rectum. Some people find it necessary to use a lubricant, which should be plant-based. Vitamin E or olive oil are fine lubricants.

8. Open stopper.

9. Let water flow in slowly. Too much water, too quickly, can be counterproductive; small amounts of water entering slowly provide deeper cleansing. If you cramp up, stop the flow and take a deep breath.

10 When you feel the urge to have a bowel movement, stop the flow of water, get up and sit on the toilet.

11 Once you feel that you have emptied your bowels, lie back down on the towel on your left side.

12 Repeat until enema bag is empty.

13 Once the enema bag is empty, you are through. Rinse your enema bag and hang up, allowing the tube to drain.

If you've never done an enema, this is really not as scary as it sounds. It is important to use distilled water and to limit the volume to 1 quart. If you do this, you can actually do enemas twice a day safely without disrupting your body, and yet help those age spots go away faster. Again, once your face is clear, you can maintain a schedule of once every week or two to have a clear complexion.

If you have a colon that is "lazy," which means that you don't feel an immediate bowel movement, add one tablespoon of lemon juice to the water. If you have a severe skin condition or rash, you can take an enema twice a day.

Figure 6. Example of old-style enema bag

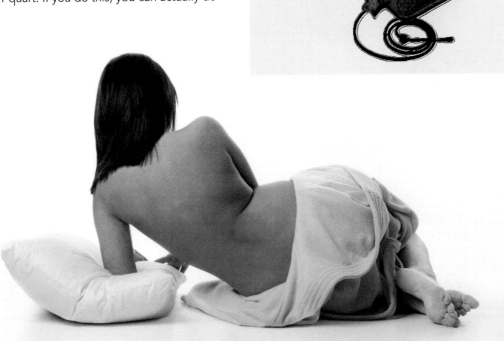

Further comments on why enemas work

If enemas are not currently part of your daily hygienic routine, you may have all kinds of reservations and concerns. As stated above, an enema is perfectly safe if executed in the way it has been described here. Dr. Daniels was taught in medical school that enemas were deadly and should never be done. After medical school, Dr. Daniels found out that these deadly enemas were extreme. They travelled too far into the colon, the temperature was too high, and the volume of water used too great (3H enemas: High, Hot, and a Helluva lot). The enema described here is very safe because it doesn't travel high into the colon, it uses only a quart of water in volume, and the water is warm to the touch.

It may help further to know why enemas work so well for removing age spots. When waste is stuck tenaciously to the inside of the wall of the intestines, some of it will get absorbed into the mucosal layer of the intestinal wall, and the blood will then pick that up. That is, the high concentration of waste on one side of the intestinal wall will

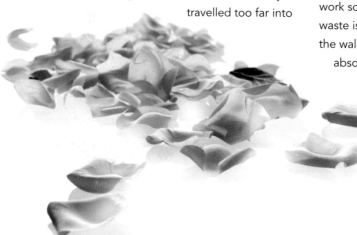

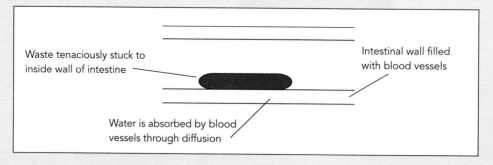

Figure 7. Waste on wall of intestine

Waste tenaciously stuck to inside wall of intestine

Intestinal wall filled with blood vessels

Water is absorbed by blood vessels through diffusion

diffuse down a concentration gradient into the intestinal wall, and then into blood vessels of the intestinal wall. This waste-laden blood is then carried to the skin, and some of the waste leaks out through the small blood capillaries in the dermis and becomes visible as an age spot. Knowing the origin of age spots makes you want to say, "Yuck!" No kidding. Hence, the enemas.

The enema reverses the flow of this chemical gradient of waste from the skin into the blood, then to the colon, and finally into the toilet where it belongs. The enemas help to dislodge the waste from the intestinal walls more efficiently than just normal bowel movements since you flush your colon with distilled water. The mucous of the intestinal wall suddenly has a low concentration of waste, the waste

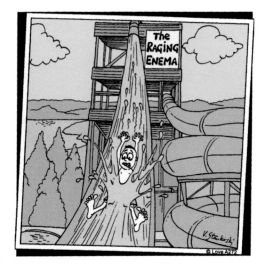

reverses direction from the skin into the toilet, and age spots begin to fade. So, an enema is a very logical, safe, and cost-effective way to remove age spots.

Figure 8. Chemical gradients of waste

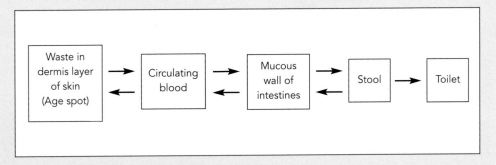

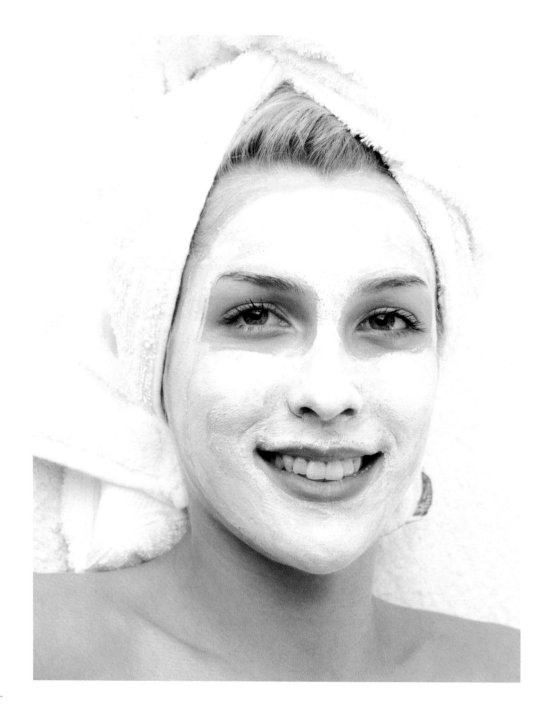

7.

Important Practices for Beautiful Skin: Facials

Let's say you are doing the best you can to be healthy and beautiful: you eat a WFPB diet, fast once a week, eat only one or two meals a day, drink the Green Drink, drink plenty of distilled water, do the enemas on a regular schedule, and maintain a positive outlook. So, you've done the best you can. You may be a little shy of perfection, but you have made changes. You have seen results, but would like to see quicker results, or more improvement. Or let's say you have a big date or a wedding to attend and you are eager to look your best. If any of the above applies to you, the facial is your salvation. *If you are adhering to the program described above, over time, you will not need a facial.* The facial is truly an intervention that becomes necessary when you have made your best effort, but are not able to do everything perfectly. The facial can bridge the gap between what you know you should do and what you actually do.

Dr. Daniels developed her own facial over years of going to spas and getting facials herself, reading Ayuervedic and Japanese beauty books, and experimentation at home. One philosophy behind her facial is not to put anything on the face that you wouldn't eat. If you wouldn't put it on your plate, then don't put it on your face! This is critical because the face absorbs material just as if you had eaten it. So, if you would not put a spoon in your moisturizer jar and eat it, or use it as an ingredient in a dish you would serve to your family, then you should not put it on your face. As we discussed earlier, chemicals that you put in your mouth are absorbed into your blood and reach your skin where they are deposited. When you put these chemicals on your skin, they are absorbed by your skin cells into the blood, and therefore into the body. Furthermore, some chemicals can enter skin cells immediately, creating visible deposits (age spots/blemishes), and can worsen the skin conditions you are trying to improve. And again, makeup can damage your skin to the point that you are embarrassed to show your face in public without applying makeup. It's a vicious cycle—but it can be broken.

Mother Earth magazine reports:

> The Environmental Working Group (EWG) found that 80% of the products they tested were contaminated with one or more substances linked to cancer and other health concerns. A recent EWG study of 15,000 cosmetics found that 22% of them were contaminated with 1,4-dioxane, which the U.S. Environmental Protection Agency classifies as a probable human carcinogen, and a known animal carcinogen. The Campaign for Safe Cosmetics (**www.safe-cosmetics.org**) says many of these chemicals are easily absorbed into the body because they're applied directly to your skin. And while the chemicals in any single product may not be a concern, repeated exposure from a variety of sources can be detrimental to your health. EWG (**www.ewg.org**) has a searchable database called Skin Deep (**www.cosmetics-database.com**), to help consumers choose better, safer personal care products [including natural and organic items].[14]

Dr. Daniels never wears any makeup. For very special occasions, Dr. Ray will wear lip gloss and eye liner made from edible products. If you choose to wear makeup sparingly, buy your makeup from local health food stores. Be sure to request an ingredient list first to find healthy products with edible ingredients, and check the database mentioned above.

Dr. Daniels' Natural Beauty Facial

Remove any makeup before doing a facial. Apply castor oil and gently remove with soft tissue or cloth and simply wipe the makeup off. Note that you don't have to worry about the myth that you rub in an upward direction to prevent skin sagging. Diet and hydration are key, not what direction you rubbed your skin during a brief facial.

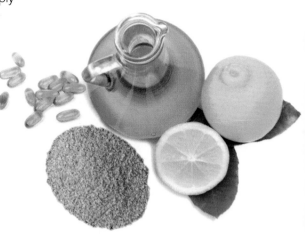

Here is an explanation of the ingredients used in the facial. Note that they are all edible and thus safe for your face. In fact, you want the nutrients to be absorbed by the skin.

Vitamin C will help kill bacteria on the skin and breaks up sebum—the greasy, waxy deposits. The scientific literature also shows that vitamin C enhances collagen production and repair when used topically. Vitamin C is an antioxidant that acts as a scavenger of free radicals, so it can decrease fine wrinkles and age spots. Vitamin C has also been promoted for topical prevention of skin damage caused by UV radiation.[15] Sun block is often recommended for prevention of UV damage to the skin. Sun block has the disadvantage of blocking valuable rays that promote vitamin D production and prevent breast cancer, arthritis, and osteoporosis. Using topical vitamin C may provide UV protection without sacrificing the benefits of vitamin D.

Rice bran is created by removing the "brown layer" of brown rice to create white rice. It has B vitamins, minerals, and fiber. The grittiness from the fiber exfoliates dead cells, diminishes blemishes on the skin, and removes the sebum and waste loosened by the vitamin C treatment. Dermabrasion is the term used to describe the removal of the top layer of skin. This process is proven to be a good and safe method to treat the scars of acne.[16] Microdermabrasion is a popular cosmetic procedure for skin rejuvenation that is achieved by mechanical abrasion of the skin at a superficial level. Small crystals are used to remove cells in this procedure. It has been shown to improve fine wrinkles, dullness, pigmentation, large pores, yellowness, and increase brightness.[17] Rice bran is the consistency of sand when it is dry. It is mildly-abrasive and can be expected to yield benefits similar to microdermabrasion. Some skin cells are removed as you gently rub your face with the softened rice bran mixture.

The scientific literature shows that with dermabrasion, benefits are seen when the top layer of cells is removed, even when no nutrients are provided. Rice bran removes cells in a similar fashion, with the added benefit of nourishing the skin with B vitamins, vitamin E, and minerals. The noticeable difference is that it helps to "plump up" the cells, which makes the wrinkles less apparent. Each time you do a facial, wrinkles diminish and your youthful appearance is restored.

Lemon soaks up the toxins while the bioflavonoids are absorbed, and this fortifies the cells so that they are not so fragile. The lemon also has a bleaching action on age spots and acne, and acts as an astringent, bringing the skin cells closer together. You will pull out toxins and wastes that were loosened by the vitamin C and rice bran, and "seal" the pores. It also tones and nourishes your skin. Studies show that topical application of citrus flavonoids inhibits sebum production in hamsters. This same mechanism may explain the beneficial effect of the lemon on acne.[18]

Grapeseed Oil (or *Jojoba oil* if you are over 40) is used to moisturize your skin. The oil takes away the tight feeling after the lemon step, but preserves the taut and silky smooth surface that was achieved.

ITEMS NEEDED:

- 1 WASHCLOTH

- WARM WATER

- 1 HAIR-BAND OR BANDANA TO PULL HAIR BACK

- 1 HAND TOWEL TO DRAPE OVER YOUR CLOTHES
  TO PROTECT THEM
  (YOU MIGHT OPT TO DO YOUR FACIAL IN THE
  SHOWER. BE SURE TO RINSE SHOWER CAREFULLY
  WHEN YOU ARE DONE TO PREVENT BACTERIAL
  GROWTH.)

- LIQUID VITAMIN C

- 1 TBS. RICE BRAN

- 1 LEMON CUT INTO WEDGES WITH JUICES SOME-
  WHAT SQUEEZED OUT. CUT LEMON TO HAVE MAXI-
  MUM EXPOSURE TO WHITES OF THE LEMON RIND

- 2 TBS. OF ORGANIC GRAPESEED OIL
  (JOJOBA OIL IF YOU ARE OVER 40)

FACIAL STEPS:

- Drape your clothes and pull hair back with
  headband.

- Rub the liquid vitamin C onto your face
  and neck, making sure to avoid the eyes.
  Wait 1–5 minutes before the next step.

- Add warm water to the rice bran and make
  a paste with about 2 tablespoons of the
  warm water. Wait a minute or two for it to
  soften so it will be gentler on your skin. It is
  not necessary to rinse off the vitamin C
  before applying the rice bran. Gently rub
  the paste into your skin and massage to
  exfoliate and nourish the skin. Do less rub-
  bing over areas like the cheeks and forehead where the skin is naturally
  thinner. Wait several minutes while the nutri-
  ents are absorbed.

- Squeeze the juice
  from the lemon.
  Press the pulp against
  your skin. Use circular motions. You will feel
  a tingling sensation. The tingling is the
  astringent action of the lemon tightening
  your skin and removing wrinkles, so don't
  rush this. Leave lemon juice on for 3–5
  minutes. When Dr. Daniels' wrinkles were
  especially severe, she left the lemon on
  overnight. You may use the edge of the
  lemon as a "razor" and remove the rice
  bran from your face. Do this cautiously as
  essential oils are released and may irritate
  your skin. The lemon also has a bleaching
  action.

- Place your washcloth in very warm water.
  Then squeeze most of the water out and
  place it over your face. Press it gently on
  your face and keep it on until it cools. Then
  use the damp cloth to remove lemon pulp
  and rice bran particles from face. Rinse the

cloth in warm water and wipe again. It may require several rinses to get all of the particles off your face.

- Finish with grapeseed or Jojoba oil; put a few drops on your hands, then spread it gently on your face. This will not plug up your pores because you have already sealed the pores with lemon as an astringent. Blot off excess oil with a clean dry towel.

As long as you feel comfortable when you do this, you may do it safely once a day for about a week, and then cut back to once or twice a week to maintain. If you have any discomfort, wait two days before repeating, or skip the step that causes discomfort.

SHORTCUTS:

Sometimes you only have a few minutes in the morning before you have to rush out the door. What do you do? Just wipe your face with a damp cloth, apply the organic oil and then wipe the excess oil from your face and go! If you have a little more time, you can do any one of the steps prior to the rinse and oil step—that is either the vitamin C, or the rice bran, or the lemon wedge step.

VARIATIONS:

1 DRY SKIN: If you have very dry skin and you have no acne or infections on your skin, then you can actually use avocado instead of organic oil. The avocado is not a uniform fruit. You want to use the more

oily green part next to the avocado skin, rub it on your skin, and leave for a minute. Remove excess to leave your face with a beautiful glow.

2 ACNE AND OILY SKIN: You can substitute the rice bran with finely ground up red lentils. It is important to grind up the lentils to a powder-like consistency and not use any larger bits that will damage the skin. Also, instead of massaging it in, it is better to pat it on and let it dry slightly on the face. This step pulls out excess oils. If the smell is too bothersome, you can use some fresh squeezed orange juice instead of water to mix with the lentils. Then gently wipe off the lentils and throw into the toilet for easy disposal.

3 AGE SPOTS: In the spring time, you can slice the stem of dandelions to get to the white sap inside. Put this sap directly on individual age spots. If you can, let it stay on overnight. Gently peel it off the next day (or it will come off with your facial) and the age spot will get lighter.

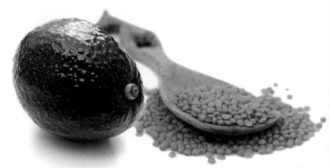

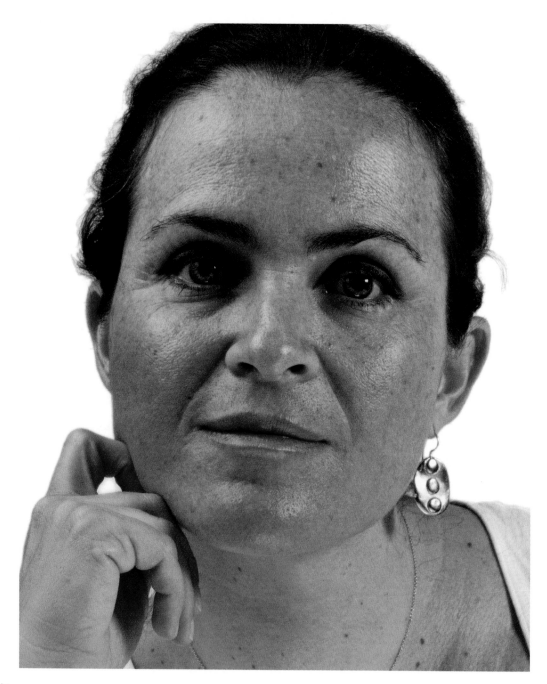

8

Important Practices for Beautiful Skin: Reading Your Face

Learning to read your face will allow you to tweak your beauty program and get the best results. You may find it easier to focus on one set of wrinkles at a time. Let's examine the different lines people commonly have on their faces, what they mean, and how to get rid of them.

Horizontal lines

Many women now have horizontal lines across their forehead. One possible explanation for these lines is that you have waste in your intestines, usually the colon; and the deeper the lines you have, the more waste has accumulated. The most expeditious way to get rid of these lines is to do a series of enemas. After ten enemas or so, you will notice those lines have substantially decreased.

Vertical liver lines

There are two short vertical lines that can appear between the eyebrows. People may call them "worry lines." In reality, these lines indicate that the liver is clogged up and is

not removing toxins properly from the body. The great news is that these lines are not permanent—you can actually get rid of them by doing liver flushes as explained in Appendix II. The deeper your lines, the more flushes you should do—generally, once a month or less. You will notice an increased sense of well-being within several days after doing a liver flush, and your lines will go away in a period of several months.

If your liver lines are not very deep or you want to prevent them, you can use milk thistle daily. The active part of this plant is the seed. The seeds are ground up and sold in capsule form, though it's cheaper to buy the seeds and grind them up fresh for your Green Drink. Artichokes are good for energizing the liver, and you can incorporate artichokes into your diet three times a week. Dr. Daniels also recommends Newton's Homeopathic Detox drops.

Crow's feet

Everybody knows what crow's feet are—the

lines that appear at the outer corners of your eyes. These are caused by processed foods and overcooked foods. They signal the need to add more raw foods and fiber to your diet, and to remove processed and overcooked foods.

Line from nose to mouth

Call them "smile lines," but they seem to get deeper with age. These are caused by a lack of minerals and omega-3 fats in the diet. These lines can also occur in the health-conscious individual who is on a plant-based diet, but who is not getting enough minerals and omega-3 fats in a form that is readily absorbable. The addition of ¼ cup of flax seeds to the Green Drink will address this.

Puffiness or bags under eyes

You've heard that you can relieve the puffiness under your eyes by applying cucumber slices. Yes, that does work because the cucumbers draw up the fluid and get rid of the puffiness. But the puffiness is a helpful symptom meant to alert you to the real problem: sugar and refined flour products in your diet. Concentrated fruit juices, evaporated cane juice, pasta, orange juice, whole wheat products, and grains can also cause this puffiness. If you aren't sure what's causing yours, you should keep a food diary. Then, when you wake up with increased puffiness, look at your food diary from the day before. Any naturally-sweetened food, such as natural soda sweetened with grape juice, or any

grain or bread, could be the culprit. Dietary changes provide quick results within days. Even "healthy" meals, such as a Portobello vegan spinach wrap, could be causing your puffiness. The wrap is made from white flour with spinach powder. The white flour causes the puffiness. Begin to read the ingredients on all food labels. The "grams of carbohydrates per serving" is misleading. You have to read the actual ingredients label. The following ingredients can cause puffiness under the eyes, and this list is not exhaustive since new types of refined carbohydrates are being devised every day.

- evaporated cane juice

- any fruit juice

- wheat

- whole wheat

- sucrose

- glucose

- fructose

- dried fruit

- high fructose corn syrup

- honey

- agave nectar

- rice flour

- date flour

Age Spots

Age spots or dyspigmentation indicate that the blood is filled with impurities. It is easy to blame this on the liver. The truth is that there are too many chemicals and sugars in the diet. The quickest way to remedy this is to switch to a chemical-free, sugar-free diet. This means the diet should not include such things as preservatives, artificial colors, artificial flavors, or hydrogenated fats. Switching to organic foods is also helpful. This generally gets rid of 50% to 75% of the problem. Enemas and daily facials get rid of the rest. Once you get your face where you want it, it is best to do a regular face check in the mirror every 7 to 14 days and increase your motivation to adhere to your program if you find a new age spot. Don't forget that at spring-time, you can take advantage of dandelions filled with sap to remove those stubborn age spots.

Enlarged Nose and Ears

If you look closely, you can see that the nose enlargement occurs in a somewhat lumpy fashion. These lumps are filled with sebum and respond well to daily facials as described earlier. The root cause is the presence of growth hormones in the diet. Dairy, beef, and pork have naturally-occurring hormones that cause growth that is inappropriate for a human. It is important to stop eating any animal whose adult weight is greater than what you consider to be your ideal body weight. The same hormones that cause the animal to reach its larger size will also cause your ears and nose to grow beyond the bounds of beauty. It is best to eliminate meat all together. If this is not possible, eat small animals that have been raised organically.

Full Lips

Those pouty lips are a sign of constipation. While they may have been glamorized by the media, they are not desirable for health. The simplest approach here is to do enemas daily for a period of time. You will see your lips get thinner. Everyone has a different amount of thickness that is normal for them. Generally, the lips you had in your high school yearbook picture are about right.

Crease in the Ear Lobe

This is a sign of heart disease, but we don't advise that you make a mad dash for your doctor's office. However, it should motivate you to make a lifestyle change. If you are a

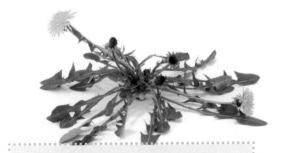

Don't forget that at spring-time, you can take advantage of dandelions filled with sap to remove those stubborn age spots.

meat eater, now is your opportunity to stop. If you do not eat meat, this is your signal to stop all of your processed foods, such as breads, crackers, or canned and packaged products. Avoiding these foods reduces the junk that can clog your arteries. Then, you need to boost your circulation. Add spices such as curry, rosemary, garlic, or cloves to your cooking. Supplements that can boost your circulation are ginkgo, hawthorn, turmeric, or cayenne, and Juice Plus+®. It is important to check with your health consultant to be sure you are using doses that are right for you.

Table 6. How to read your face diagnosis and relief summary

DESCRIPTION	CAUSE	PRESCRIPTION	RESULT EXPECTATIONS
HORIZONTAL LINES ABOVE EYEBROWS	Waste accumulated in your intestines—usually the colon	Series of enemas—once a day until you get desired results. May reduce to once a week once your goal is reached.	Improvement within a week—after about the 10th enema; dramatic results in a month.
VERTICAL LINES BETWEEN EYEBROWS	Serious problem – liver is not removing poisons	Eat artichokes 3x a week; burdock root. Take 3 milk thistle capsules 2x a day or put 1 tsp. whole milk thistle in Green Drink (less expensive choice). Take Newton's Homeopathic Detoxifier—6 drops on tongue up to 4x a day. www.newtonlabs.net	You will have a general sense of well-being in a few days. You will see lines disappearing within a few weeks and certainly by a few months.
BAGS UNDER EYES	Eating bread, sugars, store-bought juices, and pastas	Stop eating processed grains and eat more green vegetables.	Mild cases will go away in 24 hours; severe ones may take 2–7 days.
BLUE CIRCLES UNDER EYES	Bread and dairy in diet	Green Drink with milk thistle—1 tsp. Stop dairy and bread. You need a liver cleanse. See Liver Flush in Appendix II.	May take up to 7 days.

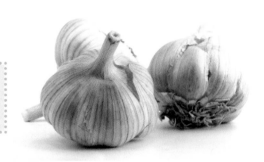

Adding spices such as curry, rosemary, garlic, or cloves to your cooking boosts your circulation.

DESCRIPTION	CAUSE	PRESCRIPTION	RESULT EXPECTATIONS
THICK, OVERLY-FULL LIPS	Constipation	You need to clean your colon. You need to do enemas.	Within 24 hours. Once colon is clean, excess fluid will leave the lips.
AGE SPOTS	Your liver is not filtering toxins or toxins are adhering to the walls of the bowel.	Drink more water. Take 3 capsules of activated charcoal with water at bedtime. You need enemas.	Most people notice improvement within 2 weeks.
CROW'S FEET	Too much cooked and processed food!	Eat more raw green vegetables. Green Drink. Facial.	If you do facials as well as dietary changes, you will notice a difference in days.
LINES AROUND LIPS, NOSE TO MOUTH	Not enough minerals and omega-3 fats being absorbed.	¼ cup ground flax seeds + 1 cup distilled water. Stir and drink.	Improvement in 1 to 2 weeks.
BIG EARS AND NOSE GETTING A BULB WITH AGE	Hormones in animal products cause your ears and nose to continue to grow!	Eliminate dairy products and meat.	It takes about a month to see change.
CREASE IN THE EAR	Serious—indicates heart disease.	Seriously need to change your diet to WFPB and eliminate all animal products, processed food, salt, and oil in diet.	Takes 2 months to see change.

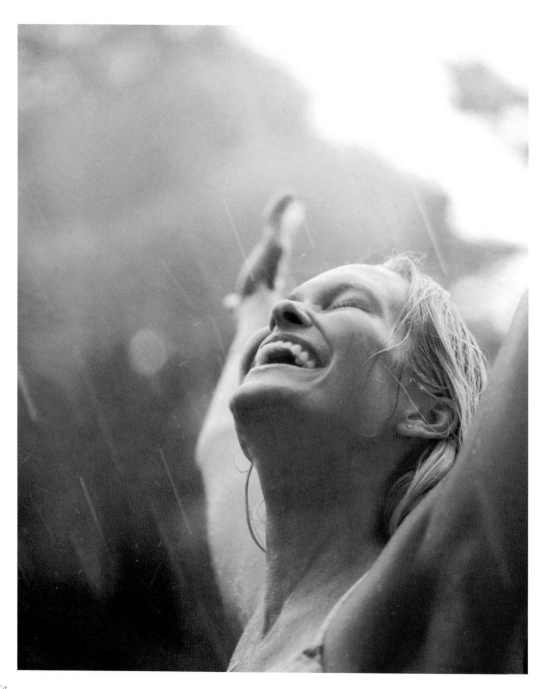

9.

Important Practices for Beautiful Skin: Sleep and Emotional Well-being

Getting plenty of sleep and taking a light-hearted approach to life will enhance your beauty. Sleep helps you regenerate the skin as well as the rest of the body. It also helps you to let go of negative emotions. If you've ever had the experience of going to bed early after a "bad day" and managing to get plenty of sleep, then you've probably experienced feeling a lot better the next day. Hence the phrase, "The sun will come out tomorrow." The resilience of your emotional state after a good night of sleep will reflect on the resilience of your skin. On the other hand, you might have experienced your emotional state after a night of partying and staying up late. Then, looking in the mirror is not that encouraging either.

Also, it is much easier to enjoy all the great blessings that being beautiful will bring into your life when you are well rested. The body uses sleep to cleanse physically and emotion-

ally. When a person is hydrated, eating well, and doing enemas, they will naturally sleep better; and all their efforts will accelerate the rejuvenation process of the skin. On the other hand, being toxic actually causes insomnia, and this can lead to a vicious cycle of not sleeping, and not looking or feeling good.

"Early to bed, early to rise" will certainly enhance beauty. Dr. Daniels advises women to get to bed by 10:00 P.M. Earlier is better. From her study of Chi gong, she learned that each hour of sleep before midnight is worth two hours of sleep after midnight. Theoretically, it is better to go to bed at 9:00 P.M. and get up at 5:00 A.M., than to go to bed at 1:00 A.M. and get up at 9:00 A.M. This type of sleep is also good for the mind. But we acknowledge that this is a lot of sleep, and not everyone can manage it. If you can, it is very helpful. Realistically, if you find yourself short on sleep, it is important for you to set aside several days a month to catch up on your sleep. In other words, sleep for 12 to 16 hours a day for about 3 days to make up for missed sleep. And never pass up a chance to nap!

In addition to sleep, having a spiritual or relaxation practice is important if you want to look your best and feel healthy and happy. Yoga, meditation, prayer, and journal writing are just a few ways that you can practice letting go of the negative emotions that weigh you down. Anger, resentment, hostility, and grief all take a serious toll on health and happiness. They will also add wrinkles to your face. You can't look good if you feel hurt or upset. This is a topic deserving its own book (and indeed there are many books written on just this thing), but it's worth mentioning that feeling relaxed, rested, and peaceful will go a long way toward helping you look youthful.

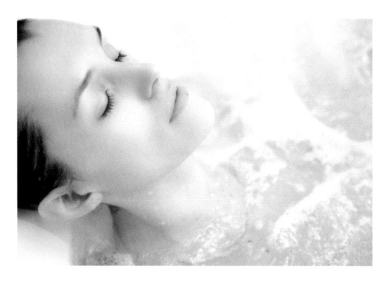

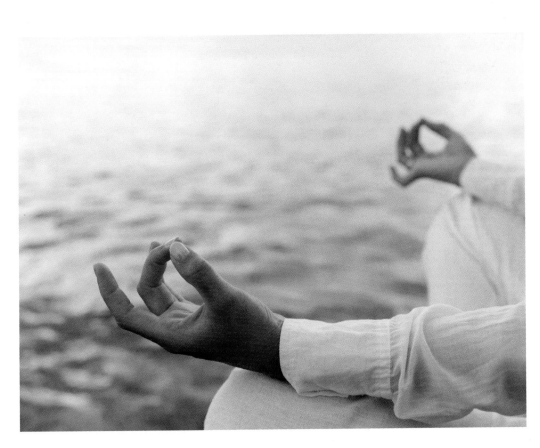

10.

Hair, Hair, Hair and No Hair

There are lots of different types of hair on the human body, but most people are only interested in increasing the amount of hair on their head. When Dr. Daniels first started working with people who said they wanted lots of hair, using natural methods, she thought, "No problem. Hair is just minerals." Two foods that are rich in minerals are black strap molasses and kelp powder, which is ground up seaweed.

So, she said to one willing patient, "Well, I can't guarantee it will work but give this a try: 2 tablespoons a day of black strap molasses (must be <50 calories per tablespoon) and 1 teaspoon of kelp powder. You have my permission to get this down any way which works for you, especially the kelp powder." Her patient tried it and was thrilled with the resultant thick hair that was growing so well. For a while, this formula helped many of her patients grow hair, and they thought that Dr. Daniels was indeed quite brilliant.

One day a new patient came in wanting to grow more hair. She was given the formula and about a month later returned with extra hair growing on her forehead. While this for-

mula does indeed help your hair grow, it can also lead to some unwanted facial fuzz!

There are several other challenges with hair:

1. Hair growth needs to be gender appropriate. Women don't want beards, and men don't want to lose their beards.

2. Results with hair growth should happen in less than 4 weeks. As a well-trained medical doctor, Dr. Daniels was familiar with other treatments that take anywhere from 6 to 24 weeks before you can see effects.

3. Losing hair pigmentation or graying was another challenge to consider. Certainly genetic predisposition plays a role, since some people tend to gray sooner than others. The other factor again is minerals—selenium, copper, and trace minerals. Not getting enough minerals could be simply the result of your not eating enough mineral-rich foods, or because your intestines are not absorbing minerals like they used to. A lifetime of eating poorly can create a barrier layer on the lining of your small intestines that interferes with the absorption

of minerals and other nutrients. This is why the same diet that was adequate in nutrients at one point in your life becomes inadequate 20 years later. You are no longer absorbing the nutrients as well as you did 20 years ago. Hair pigment is easier to reverse than hair loss.

To slow down graying

Let's say you have a few gray hairs and you are plucking them out and it's not too serious, but you would like to hold the line—maybe you have fewer than 100 gray hairs. Taking a whole food based nutritional supplement rich in phytonutrients (plant nutrients) and minerals might be a worthwhile investment in order to increase antioxidants and minerals in the blood, and provide many other health benefits.[h]

Absorption of nutrients in the gut may be another issue. The simplest quick fix for the absorption issue is the Green Drink. It provides minerals as well as fiber that scrubs the small intestines and gets the walls clean enough so that they will absorb more minerals and help the hair to get its pigment back. Note that the part of the hair that is already gray will not turn back to its natural pigment. Only the new part of the hair growing from the root (hair follicle) will be pigmented.

More Serious Graying

Let's say you have more than 100 gray hairs. One formulation that Dr. Daniels likes

---

[h] Juice Plus+® is a whole food based nutritional supplement with clinical research showing many health benefits, including the bioavailability of trace minerals such as selenium. Anecdotally, it has helped some people slow down gray hair and balding. www.juiceplus.com

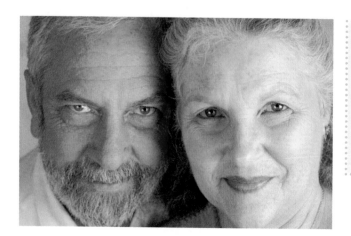

A lifetime of eating poorly can create a barrier layer on the lining of your small intestines that interferes with the absorption of minerals and other nutrients—one factor in graying.

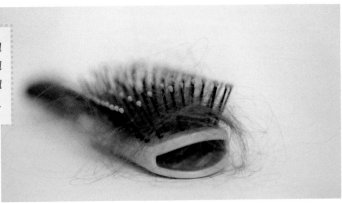

is called Fo-Ti, also known as He Shou Wu.[i] Research shows that the major side effect of taking Fo-Ti everyday is that you can expect to live about 20 years longer—it extends your life expectancy. If you have lived too long already, then stop taking your Fo-Ti! For men, it will also increase your libido. Neither the hair nor the other benefits will be achieved instantly. It works over time. In order to get results, however, large quantities of Fo-ti are needed. We have created our own proprietary formulation of concentrated Fo-ti with minerals and white tea, and only two to four capsules a day are necessary to see results (please check resources in the back of the book). The other option is to find a local Chinese pharmacy and take 12-14 pills a day, and also take additional minerals. Colloidal minerals and other liquid minerals are useful for treating gray hair and, to some

extent, baldness. The liquid mineral dosage for grayness is four tablespoons per day (¼ cup) or twice the recommended dose on the bottle—use the amount that is the smaller of the two. This can be consumed in water or ¼ cup of fruit juice.

Thinning hair and baldness

To address baldness, the number one issue to address is lack of circulation to the scalp; when the hair loses its blood supply, it falls out. The next issue to consider with baldness is hormones. Dr. Daniels doesn't subscribe to the theory that testosterone causes baldness. She believes that there are intermediate metabolites that are present in both men and women that bind to the hair follicles and cause them to go dormant. Dr. Daniels believes that the source of these metabolites

---

[i] "He" refers to the family name of the Chinese doctor who discovered the power of the herb. "Shou Wu" has two meanings in Mandarin. The words refer to gray hair turning black, and on a deeper level it means the regaining of youth.

is animal products and processed foods. In *The China Study*, T. Colin Campbell found an association between increased animal protein in the diet and baldness in men.[19]

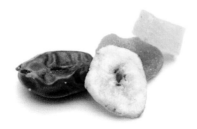

There are two ways to address the lack of circulation issue. The first way is rather tedious but quite effective, and that is to simply put all ten fingertips on the head and vigorously rub for at least five minutes a day. The way to rub is by keeping your head still and moving your scalp, almost as if it's a hairpiece that

One effective way to address the lack of circulation in the scalp is to simply put all ten fingertips on the head and vigorously rub for at least five minutes a day. This is going to re-stimulate blood flow to the follicles and cause your hair to grow.

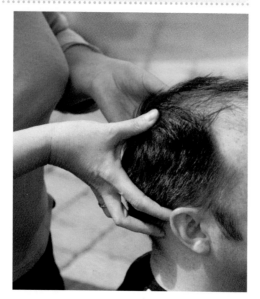

you are moving around. This is going to re-stimulate blood flow to the follicles and cause your hair to grow. If you do only this and nothing else, you will have some success. But if you combine this with the Fo-Ti and the colloidal minerals, you will get quicker results.

There is a dietary component to balding. Concentrated sweets, meats, or oils seem to make balding worse. What is a concentrated sweet? Presuming that anyone reading this book is already a health-minded person, then what should be mentioned are foods such as dried fruit, or fruit-pureed into a nut ball, or power bars with dried fruit in them. Eating these nice, vegan, raw treats will adversely affect your hair. Next, let's talk about these great vegan recipes that call for a lot of oil. As it turns out, many people who are on raw, vegan diets experience incredible thinning of their hair because of unhealthful oils in their food.

What if you are not a health nut? In addition to the dietary changes above, you need to at least switch to meats that have no hormones added, and to eating meat or animal products from animals that don't grow any bigger than people, such as chickens. In other words, beef, pork, and dairy have got to go. If you are going to eat chicken, make sure that there are no hormones or animal products added either to the chicken itself or to the chicken feed. This is an important nuance because a lot of the chickens in the USA are being fed ground-up cows, and they don't count that as a hormone additive! So, switch to organic, vegetarian-fed chickens. Cage-free is best, if possible.

Drinking enough water is also important since dehydration will lessen the circulation of blood to the hair follicle. It is a waste of your efforts to take minerals or Fo Ti if the blood is not being circulated to the scalp.

Now, let's say you've made these dietary changes—which are not as extensive as those for beautiful skin—and you would still like to further enhance your hair growth. The most effective treatment Dr. Daniels has ever used for hair loss is called "small willow flower." This comes as an extract in a 2-oz. bottle and you will want to order at least two bottles.[j] Take two full droppers in ¼ cup of water and

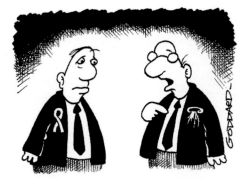

"It's for hair loss awareness".

drink this twice a day. If you have any hair, you will notice first that the hair is thicker. Around week three, the growth becomes exuberant. This will get rid of baldness. Even if you have a bald spot or receding hairline, you will actually see hair growing and restoring hairlines. It, interestingly enough, has the side benefit of improving prostate conditions.

The other interesting observation that Dr. Daniels has made is that men who have prostate cancer tend to be bald.

[j] See Resources.

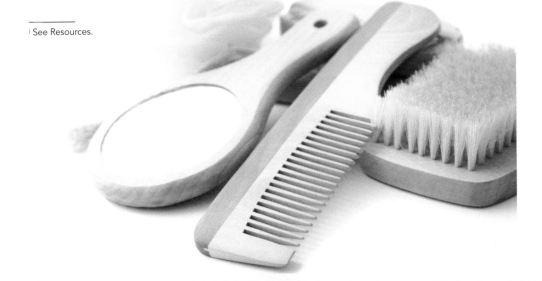

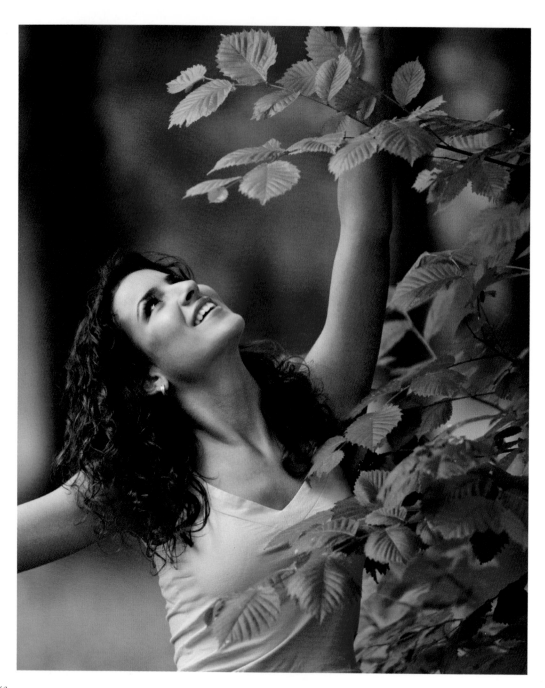

11.

Beautiful You, Beautiful Planet

Lately there has been increased awareness and concern about the effects of global warming and the over-consumption of natural resources by humans. It is commonplace now for families to reuse and recycle, to carpool or bike or walk when possible, and to conserve water and energy in our daily lives. Low energy light bulbs, water-reducing shower heads, and hybrid automobiles are just a few of the inventions that we are able to utilize to reduce our carbon footprints and to try to impact the Earth as little as possible.

These are laudable steps that people can feel good about taking. Of course, the fewer chemicals we use on our faces, the less we support the making of these chemicals, and the associated pollution and gas emissions. Yet, the most frightening cause of global warming and land degradation remains unknown and unaddressed by most people. Nothing affects our impact upon Mother Earth so much as factory farming practices, and our continued consumption of meat and other animal products. Following a WFPB diet will not only help you to look beautiful—it's the biggest thing that you as an individual can do to help keep the *Earth* beautiful.

The unnecessary use of important natural resources

Did you know that it takes between 2,000 and 5,000 gallons of water to produce one pound of beef? (The number varies based on location of the livestock).[20] Conversely, it takes 23 gallons of water to produce one pound of tomatoes. It takes 49 gallons to produce one pound of apples. While many Americans are willing to forgo watering their lawns in the summer, we're each consuming *tens of thousands of gallons of water* every week just by following the standard American diet. Turning off the tap when you brush your teeth or taking a shorter shower is nothing compared to the thousands of gallons of water required to feed each meat-eating human. Just think about that: more than 2,000 gallons of water are used to produce a single pound of meat. That's a whole lot of long showers and lawn watering.

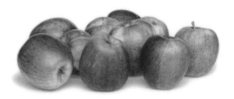

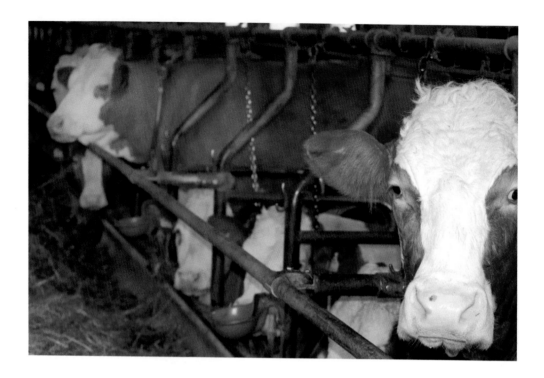

The thing is, water is not a renewable resource. Current human water consumption is draining aquifers and drying up wells worldwide. There's no invention out there that's going to allow us to replace the world's water. When it's gone, it's gone. Following a WFPB diet is by far the best thing that you can do to conserve water.

Just as startling as the waste of water are the fuel use and pollution that are caused by the meat and dairy industries. The production of one pound of beef uses 16 times the amount of gasoline that is required to produce one pound of vegetables and rice. That same pound of beef is responsible for an estimated 24 times the amount of greenhouse gas emissions as that pound of vegetables and rice.

It's not just the resources that are used to grow livestock that we need to be concerned with. Animal waste is an appalling cause of soil contamination, land degradation, and illness. A single cow produces 14.6 tons of manure annually. That's the equivalent size and weight of approximately 10 automobiles. A single hog produces 16.7 tons of manure annually. Now multiply those tons of manure by the millions of livestock alive at any given point, and you come up with a staggering figure. USA livestock produces close to 900 million tons of manure annually.

Ok, so that's a lot of waste. So what? Doesn't animal waste turn into fertilizer, which helps soil content and aids plant growth? Actually, no. Livestock produce 130 times the amount of solid waste that humans do.[21] But while the disposal of human waste is tightly regulated and controlled, the same is not always true of animal waste. Trillions of pounds of untreated excrement are produced each year, and where does it go? Well, it's either sprayed over crop fields, or left in huge "lagoons." Neither of these options is a good solution; both produce run off that kills fish and other wildlife, destroys soil, and contaminates water. It's far more waste than can be absorbed by the earth, which means that it becomes pollution of the worst kind.

A Scripps Howard analysis of a Senate Agricultural Committee report had this to say about animal waste:

[It's] untreated and unsanitary, bubbling with chemicals and diseased. . . . It goes onto the soil and into the water that many people will, ultimately, bathe in and wash their clothes with and drink. It is poisoning rivers and killing fish and making people sick. . . . Catastrophic cases of pollution, sickness, and death are occurring in areas where livestock operations are concentrated. . . . Every place where the animal factories have located, neighbors have complained of falling sick.[22]

The livestock industry is one of the largest contributors to environmental damage worldwide, inflicting deforestation, air and water pollution, land degradation, loss of topsoil, climate change, the overuse of resources including oil and water, and loss of biodiversity. If you're an environmentalist, or just someone who wants their children and grandchildren to have a healthy planet to live on, the mandate is clear: follow a plant-based diet.

It's not just the resources that are used to grow livestock that we need to be concerned with. Animal waste is an appalling cause of soil contamination, land degradation, and illness.

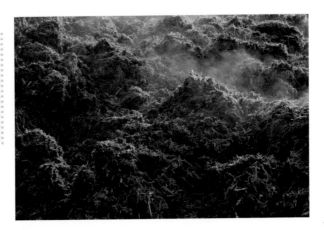

Animal suffering

Entire tomes have been penned on this topic, and while pushing an animal rights agenda isn't the goal of this book, it's worth saying a few words—it may be time for us to reconsider our choice to support the horrors inflicted upon livestock that are raised for human consumption.

> The world must create five billion vegans in the next several decades, or triple its total farm output without using more land.
>
> —Dennis Avery, Director of the Centre for Global Food Issues

So why do we eat meat? Because we think we need it as a source of protein. While we won't go into great detail about this issue here, we should say that it is impossible to be deficient in protein on a WFPB diet. Plants carry out photosynthesis and do work—thus they are full of enzymes, which are protein. Calorie for calorie, a plant-based diet has as much protein as an animal-based diet.[23] A recent study also showed that eating plants is better for preserving lean mass, and it may be because plant protein is less acidic to the body.

> The typical American diet is rich in protein. . . and other acid-producing foods. In general, such diets generate tiny amounts of acid each day. With aging, a mild but slowly increasing metabolic "acidosis" develops, according to the researchers.[24]

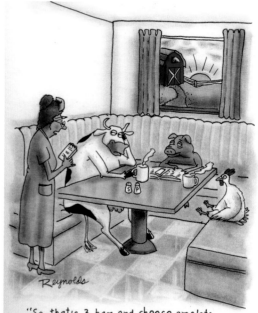

"So, that's 3 ham and cheese omelets . . . one order without cheese, one without ham, and another without eggs."

Still not convinced? Just look at a stallion—with all its beautiful muscles—and consider that this beautiful animal got that way from eating grass! While you don't have to chew on grass, consider that the preservation of lean mass through a WFPB diet makes for a *beautiful body* as well. And it is not lost on us that the color of the Green Drink makes one think that it might as well be ground up grass!

Let's *reconsider:* what is beauty? In the beginning of the book, we declared:

Beauty is when the cells in your body radiate a message of health to the world. This radiance is universally attractive. You feel good about yourself, and others feel good about being around you. Beauty is an "inside job!"

In light of this chapter, we might redefine beauty from a global perspective to say:

Beauty is when the cells in your body radiate a message of health to the world, and the world radiates back at you. Our radiance and the earth's radiance are universally attractive. Inner beauty and outer beauty come together in Mother Earth and her inhabitants.

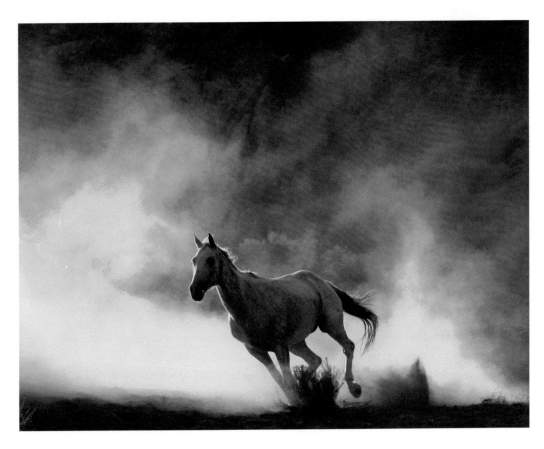

Appendix I

If You Are Going to Eat Meat

If you are going to eat meat, you will need to follow the guidelines below. It's a bit like safe sex: if you are going to do it, protect yourself!

1. Make sure you drink even more water than what we are recommending in Table 5.

2. Never give up the Green Drink as part of your daily regimen.

3. Do not combine starches (bread, pasta) with meat in the same meal. On a WFPB diet, food combining is a nonissue. But when eating meat, it becomes a big issue.

4. Instead of bread and pasta, eat potatoes and whole grains, such as brown rice, quinoa, or millet. Wait at least two hours before eating meat.

5. Eat meat between 10:00 A.M. and 4:00 P.M., when your digestion is strongest and your body is most able to remove the high waste load, and you will be less likely to "wear" your meat meal.

6. Eat four times the volume in vegetables as the meat you are having. Vegetables provide the fiber that absorbs the damaging chemicals in the meat. Vegetables also release the antioxidants that can protect your body from the cellular damage that meat can cause. You can order stir-fried vegetables, with fewer than usual strips of meat and more vegetables as an example of this blending.

7. Use spices to neutralize the parasites that are always present in meat. Salt and pepper are not enough to protect your good looks from the effects of meat. Recommended spices include garlic, oregano, rosemary, thyme, cloves, turmeric, cilantro, cumin, asafoetida, ginger, and cayenne pepper. Small amounts are not enough. The meat should be smothered with spices. Curried goat or blackened fish are two examples of this natural neutralization.

8. The concept of a "lean meat" is urban mythology; fish, poultry, and red meat all have similar amounts of high cholesterol and saturated fat. The high-fat content constricts the arteries for up to 6 hours. Use whole food based supplementation[k] which has been clinically shown to reduce this negative effect on the arteries.[25]

---

k www.juiceplus.com

THE ULTIMATE LIVER FLUSH

Let's say you have countless age spots and you are really committed to getting rid of them quickly. Then you need to do a liver flush. The health benefit is that you will clear your congested liver, and it will become a much more effective filter for your blood. This means that your liver will do a much better job of removing the chemicals that cause age spots. This also reduces the amount of antioxidants your body needs to neutralize these chemicals. These nutrients will then be available to enhance your beauty instead. You cannot rush any of the following steps, including the re-feeding process, if you want to minimize your discomfort and maximize your benefit. Best of luck for the brave!

Preparation for the liver flush: *In order to minimize the detoxification symptoms of the liver flush, please follow a WFPB Beauty diet, proper hydration, and at least weekly enemas for 30 days before attempting the liver flush. This is important.*

Day 1-4

Drink ½ gallon to 1 gallon of apple juice each day. The apple juice softens stones; hard irregular stones can hurt to pass. Realistically you want to eat very light food—raw fruits and veggies —or just fast on the apple juice. You can also take malic acid (magnesium malate) supplements 2–3 times a day if you find it difficult to consume such volumes of apple juice.

Day 5

Eat only raw veggies in the morning, water in afternoon. At 6:00 P.M., take 1 tablespoon of Epsom salts in a pint of water. Repeat at 9:00 P.M. The raw veggies and Epsom salts clear the intestines so that the stool gets out of the way, and bile and waste can flow freely from the liver into the intestines. Skipping this step will cause the bile to go backwards up the esophagus (food pipe), and it will taste something awful. Then, this bile will get reabsorbed by the liver before it goes forward to the intestines. Skipping this step ruins the hard work you have done in the first 4 days of the liver flush.

Day 6

Fast with water—repeat Epsom salts at 3:00 P.M.

At 6:00 P.M. drink 2-4 tablespoons of olive oil (depending on body weight and tolerance), then 2 tablespoons of lemon juice. Repeat every 15 minutes for 8 doses total. Note that the last 3 doses will take a long time, and you will hate olive oil forever and may feel nauseous. But hating olive oil forever will be a good thing. It's a processed fat, and not the health food it is touted to be.

Olive oil stimulates the gall bladder to contract and release bile. Olive oil then is absorbed by the liver and flushes out the chemicals and biological waste products from the bile ducts. These substances are released into the intestines. If there is stool in the intestines blocking the bile from going forward, it will go backward causing nausea, vomiting, and a foul taste in the mouth.

Lemon juice clears your pallet and stimulates the intestines in the proper direction.

Lay on your right side and go to bed. You will experience a gentle gurgling sensation. It will feel like soft pebbles rolling around in the liver under your right rib cage. This is from the olive oil loosening the debris from the bile ducts.[1] Around 2:00 A.M., you will experience a bowel movement and stone-like debris will come out from the liver without pain.

Day 7

At 6:00 A.M., take more Epsom salts (1 tablespoon in a pint of water); you will most likely experience more debris coming out painlessly. Do a juice fast for the rest of the day.

Day 8

Eat raw fruits and veggies only for the day.

Day 9

You can now eat fruits, and raw and steamed veggies.

Dr. Daniels has done this many times—the right way and the wrong way. There is a fair amount

---

[1] There is much controversy about what kind of stones are passed during a liver flush—some say they are pre-gall bladder stones, while others whole-heartedly disagree. Nonetheless, the changes in appearance are what we are interested in here, and the liver flush does enhance beauty. It will also enhance the other efforts in your beauty regimen, such as the effectiveness of the enemas.

If by chance you've had your gallbladder removed, it is still fine to do the liver flush. Just be meticulous about the apple juice and magnesium malate supplements to help soften the stones and prevent discomfort.

of disagreement as to whether the debris that comes out is gall stones. Leaving this aside, the elimination of waste and the improvement in your looks is undeniable.

APPENDIX III

YOGIC HYDRATION

You should drink a glass of water first thing in the morning, before your feet hit the ground. Additionally, you can use water to further cleanse the body (as the ancient yogis did) as follows—but only if you are not taking any medication, if you are eating a WFPB diet, and if you have not had any alcohol the night before. Check with your health care provider if you have any doubts.

If you follow the advice of the 5,000-year-old yoga practices, the best way to use water as a *cleanser* is to drink 2–9 glasses of room-temperature water upon waking. Initially, drinking even 1 glass on an empty stomach may be uncomfortable. Again, this practice is really for people who are quite healthy and not on medication. You can start with 1 glass, and if you have trouble, try not to taste it by drinking slowly, but rather just get it down. Work your way up to even larger volumes as it feels comfortable. Remember, these are lifelong habits you are implementing.

Don't consume anything for another half hour, if possible. So drink your water first, then brush your teeth; maybe do a quick facial, or if you are following an enema regimen do that; get dressed, and work your way to the kitchen to put together your morning Green Drink. This will take up the half hour easily.

If you develop this practice, the rewards that people report include radiant skin, some weight loss, better bowel functions, reduction in headaches and joint pains, and better immune system. Remember that this practice is in addition to the regular habit of drinking water throughout the day, since you still need a great deal of water to keep your body hydrated as the day progresses.

Suggested Readings

- *The China Study* by T. Colin Campbell (BenBella Books, Inc., 2005).

- *Green for Life* by Victoria Boutenko (Raw Family Publishing, 2005).

- *Tissue Cleansing Through Bowel Management* by Bernard Jensen (Bernard Jensen International, 1981, 12th edition).

- *RAVE Diet and Eating* DVD by Mike Anderson (www.RaveDiet.com, 2004).

- *Food Revolution* by John Robbins (Conari Press, 2001).

Resources

Supplementation

- Juice Plus®—**www.JuicePlus.com** or call your Juice Plus+® distributor

- Currently we are developing more resources for beauty. So check for updates on **www.DrMitraRay.com**.

- Small Willow Flower and Fo-Ti can be ordered from 1-877-315-9880 or online at **www.DrMitraRay.com**.

- A good brand of liquid minerals is ConcenTrace® Trace Mineral Drops. **www.TraceMinerals.com**

Facials

- Look for Facial start up kits soon available on **www.DrMitraRay.com**.

Enemas

- www.EnemaBag.com/how_to_take_an_enema.html

Vita-Mix

- The Vita-Mix (**www.vitamix.com**) is an awesome blender for making green drinks, soups, and other whole food meals. We have arranged with Vita-Mix to offer our readers free shipping ($25US/$35CN). **When ordering, you must use this special code: 06-004250.**

BIBLIOGRAPHY

[1] Bradley, B., "A Fresh Face." *The Commercial Appeal*, Memphis, TN. (October 26, 2008).

[2] Choi, C.M., Berson, D.S., "Cosmeceuticals." *Seminars in Cutaneous Medicine and Surgery*, 25 (3): 163-8 (2006).

[3] Singh, M, Griffiths, C.E.M., "The use of retinoids in the treatment of photoaging." *Dermatologic Therapy*, 19(5): 297-305, (2006).

[4] Krautheim, A. Gollnick, H., "Transdermal Penetration of Topical Drugs Used in the Treatment of Acne." *Clinical Pharmacokinetics*, 42(14): 1287-1304 (2003).

[5] Helfrich, Y.R., Sachs, D.L., Voorhees, J.J., "Overview of Skin Aging and Photoaging." *Dermatology Nursing*, 20(3):177-183 (2008).

[6] Callaghan T., Wilhelm, K.P., "A review of ageing and an examination of clinical methods in the assessment of ageing skin. Part 2: Clinical perspectives and clinical methods in the evaluation of ageing skin." *International Journal of Cosmetic Science*, 30(5): 323-332 (2008).

[7] Monestier, S., Gaudy, C., Gouvernet, J., Richard, M., Grob, J., "Multiple senile lentigos of the face, a skin ageing pattern resulting from a life excess of intermittent sun exposure in dark-skinned caucasians: a case-control study." *British Journal of Dermatology*, 154(3): 438-44 (2006).

[8] Jensen, Bernard, *Tissue Cleansing Through Bowel Management*, Bernard Jensen International, 12th edition (1981).

[9] Rawlings A.V., "Ethnic skin types: are there differences in skin structure and function?" *International Journal of Cosmetic Science*, 28(2): 79-93 (2006).

[10] Monestier, S., Gaudy, C., Gouvernet, J., Richard, M., Grob, J., "Multiple senile lentigos of the face, a skin ageing pattern resulting from a life excess of intermittent sun exposure in dark-skinned caucasians: a case-control study." *British Journal of Dermatology*, 154(3): 438-44 (2006).

[11] Tehrani, R., Nash-Goelitz, A., Adams, E., Dahiya, M., and Eilers, D., "Minocycline-induced cutaneous polyarteritis nodosa." *Journal of Clinical Rheumatology*, 13(3): 146-9 (2005).

Also you can carefully read the package insert for acne medication such as Accutane.

[12] Beguin, A., "A novel micronutrient supplement in skin aging: a randomized placebo-controlled double-blind study." *Journal of Cosmetic Dermatology*, 4(4): 277-84 (2005).

[13] Liska, D.J., "The Detoxification Enzyme Systems." *Alternative Medicine Review*, 3(3): 187-98 (1998).

[14] Bloyd, S., "What's Your Makeup Made Of?" *Mother Earth News*, (August/September 27, 2008).

[15] Yu, R., Van Scott, E., "Alpha-hydroxyacids and carboxylic acids." *Journal of Cosmetic Dermatology*, 3(2): 76-87 (2004).

[16] Rivera A.E., "Acne scarring: a review and current treatment modalities." *Journal of the American Academy of Dermatology*, 59(4): 659-76 (2008).

[17] Spencer, J. M. and Kurtz, E.S., "Approaches to Document the Efficacy and Safety of Microdermabrasion Procedure." *Dermatologic Surgery*, 32(11): 1353-7 (2006).

[18] Sato, T. Takahashi, A., Kojima, M., Akimoto, N., Yano, M., Ito, A., "A citrus polymethoxy flavonoid, nobiletin inhibits sebum production and sebocyte proliferation, and augments sebum excretion in hamsters." *Journal of Investigative Dermatology*, 127(12); 2740-8 (2007).

[19] Campbell, T. Colin, *The China Study*, BenBella Books, Inc. (2005).

[20] Robbins, John, *The Food Revolution: How Your Diet Can Help Save Your Life and Our World*, Conari Press, (2001).

[21] Lang, J., "U.S. Staggers Under Weight of Waste From Farm Animals." *Scripps Howard News Service*, 26 Apr, 1998.

[22] Campbell, T. Colin, *The China Study*, BenBella Books, Inc. (2005).

[23] Dawson-Hughes B, Harris SS, Ceglia L., "Alkaline diets favor lean tissue mass in older adults." *American Journal of Clinical Nutrition*, 87(3): 662-5 (2008).

[24] Bliss, R. M., "Plant Foods for Preserving Muscle Mass." USDA Agriculture Research Service. Retrieved November 16, 2008, from USDA Agriculture Research Service: http://www.ars.usda.gov/is/pr/2008/080523.htm (May 23, 2008).

[25] Plotnick, G.D., Corretti, M.C., Vogel, R. A., Hesslink, Jr., R., Wise, J., "Effect of Supplemental Phytonutrients on Impairment of the Flow-Mediated Brachial Artery Vasoactivity After A Single High-Fat Meal." *Journal of the American College of Cardiology*, 41 (10): 1744-9 (2003).

For more information, or to order additional copies of this book
at a volume discount, contact us:

Shining Star Media
P.O. Box 383
Marysville, Washington 98270
www.DrMitraRay.com